Exclusively Pumping Breast Milk

A Guide to Providing Expressed Breast Milk for Your Baby

Stephanie Casemore

• Gray Lion Publishing •

Exclusively Pumping Breast Milk
A Guide to Providing Expressed Milk for Your Baby
by Stephanie Casemore

Published by:
Gray Lion Publishing
282 Barrett Blvd.
Napanee, Ontario Canada K7R 1G8
graylion@sympatico.ca

For orders and additional information:
www.exclusivelypumping.com
info@exclusivelypumping.com

Printed in Canada

Copyeditor: Tamala Szyman

Library and Archives Canada Cataloguing in Publication

Casemore, Stephanie, 1971-
Exclusively pumping breast milk: a guide to providing expressed breast milk for your baby / Stephanie Casemore.

ISBN 0-9736142-0-X

1. Breast milk--Collection and preservation. 2. Breast pumps.
I. Title.

RJ216.C345 2004 649'.33   C2004-904666-7

Table of Contents

Acknowledgments

I am tremendously grateful to the many people who have supported me and encouraged me while writing this book. Without you, it would never have left my computer.

Thank you to Shelley, Tamala, and Kristin for reading the early drafts of the book and giving such invaluable feedback, suggestions, and advice.

Thank you to the many women I have met online who have provided their unending support, knowledge, and experience to me both while I was pumping and while I was writing this book. The camaraderie among women who are exclusively pumping is incredible. You are truly a very special group of women.

Thank you to my husband for his constant faith, support, and encouragement. Without you, I would never have faced the cold basement during the winter where I spent many hours writing the first draft.

And most of all, thank you to my son. It was your precious life that led me down the road I am now on. We are blessed to have you in our world. I love you.

Warning — Disclaimer

This book is designed to provide information on exclusively pumping breast milk. It is sold with the understanding that the author and publisher are not engaged in providing medical or lactation advice or other professional services. The information presented in this book is based on the personal experience of the author. If you require medical or other expert assistance, you should seek the services of a competent professional. Before taking any course of action that may affect you, or your baby, it is strongly advised that you consult with a medical professional.

It is not the purpose of this book to reprint all sources of information available on the subject of lactation, breastfeeding, or exclusively pumping. You are urged to read all available material and learn as much as you can about lactation, breastfeeding, and exclusively pumping, and then modify the information to your individual needs.

Every effort has been made to make this book complete and accurate. However, there may still be mistakes, both typographical and in content. It is for this reason that this text should be used only as a general guide and not as the ultimate source of information about exclusively pumping or lactation.

The author and Gray Lion Publishing shall have neither liability nor responsibility to any person or entity with respect to any loss or damage caused, or alleged to have been caused, directly or indirectly, by the information contained in this book.

An Important Note about Individuality

It is important to begin this book by saying there is no right way to exclusively pump. Each woman is an individual and each woman will find success in a different way. There is no prescriptive method to building and maintaining your supply. There is no sure-fire method to success. What it takes is an understanding of lactation, patience, dedication, and the ability to listen to your body and understand how your body is reacting to the changes you make in your pumping routine. Yet unfortunately, even following all the guidelines and techniques recommended by other pumping mothers and knowledgeable lactation consultants, some women may still have difficulty establishing and maintaining a strong supply.

The information provided in this book is based on my experience exclusively pumping for one year, as well as the experience of many women who have also exclusively pumped with whom I communicated with over the Internet. Accept this information as guidelines that have proven successful for many women. There are women who have veered outside of these guidelines and have still been able to successfully pump long-term, and some women who have ventured away from the guidelines have not been able to establish and maintain a supply.

Introduction

Throughout my pregnancy I planned on breastfeeding. I knew that I wanted to give my baby the best I possibly could, and for me that meant providing breast milk for as long as possible. Around the beginning of my third trimester, I began to read books on the subject of breastfeeding wanting to be sure I was prepared and knowledgeable. But having the time to read the volumes of information I collected was not to be.

Thirty weeks into my pregnancy, I developed severe and sudden preeclampsia and was immediately admitted into the antenatal ward of the hospital. Within four days of being admitted, I was induced and my tiny three pound two ounce baby boy was born. Thankfully, he wasn't born with any serious complications other than his low birth weight, and, with the intention of giving him the best I could, I set out pumping since he was too small to nurse.

Initially, pumping was only intended to initiate my milk supply and ensure that I could breastfeed once my son was ready. Three weeks after his birth, I began short attempts to breastfeed him, and surprisingly, he seemed eager and ready. However, even after joining him in the hospital around the clock for almost two weeks, he was not strong enough to take full feeds by breast and continued to be fed by a nasogastric (NG) tube which is a tube fed through the nose directly into the stomach.

By the time he was thirty-seven weeks gestational age, we decided to introduce a bottle in order to get him home. Hospital policy stated that a baby could not leave the Infant Intensive Care Unit (IICU) until he or she was able to take all feeds by mouth for a 48 hour period. The importance of bringing our baby home before he fell ill in the hospital from the many viruses and bacteria lurking there was mentioned to me a number of times by different nurses. And so three weeks before his due date, we introduced the bottle and brought our tiny baby home.

Once home, life became an endless cycle of breastfeeding, bottle feeding to ensure he was receiving enough, and then pumping. On a good night, I was able to get four hours of sleep, although rarely four consecutive hours. Having been told to wake my baby every three hours to eat, I was quickly running on empty. Our breastfeeding efforts quickly deteriorated into extremely stressful experiences. My son would wail anytime I attempted to bring him to breast. He would scream and thrash and refuse to latch on. Needing to feed him, I resorted to bottle feeding in order to supplement our "failed" breastfeeding attempts. Throughout this, I continued to pump.

Eventually, in an effort of self-preservation, I decided that I would pump exclusively and feed by bottle. Once this decision was made, the stress level in the house dropped dramatically. Everyone, including my dog, seemed a little less on edge. But now I was faced with a future tied to a breast pump and no where to go for support or information about exclusively pumping.

The Internet became my best resource, and I located a number of discussion boards focusing on women who were pumping for their babies. Suddenly I was no longer alone, and I realized it was possible to pump long-term. These women became my source of expertise since these were the women doing it and proving it could be successful. Since at that time there were no available resources dedicated to exclusively pumping, women had to figure it out for themselves. Not only did the internet provide much needed support and camaraderie, it also provided a valuable forum for women who were exclusively pumping to share their experience and techniques.

I continued to work with my son to develop a latch that did not rely on the use of the nipple shield that we had begun to use while still in the hospital. A couple weeks after his due date we had success, put away the shield, and continued our efforts. Although I did not transition over to breastfeeding exclusively, my son did continue to breastfeed occasionally, often as a comfort measure and sometimes just because he was hungry. Complications with nipple soreness on my part, severe reflux on my son's part that was not diagnosed for a number of months, and his preference for the bottle nipple prevented a transition to breastfeeding. And so I pumped, happy to do it for the health of my son. I am grateful, however, that I was able to experience some aspect of breastfeeding although not the breastfeeding relationship I had expected. I exclusively pumped for just over one year and weaned by choice. After I weaned, I had enough frozen milk to feed my son expressed breast milk for another couple months.

Exclusively pumping is an option! However, many women are not aware of it or are sometimes told that it is rarely possible and that they may not maintain a supply with a pump. While it is true that not every woman will see success, many women will, and obtaining good advice about exclusively pumping is the best way to achieve this success.

I am not a medical professional. I have no background in lactation or breastfeeding support. But I did exclusively pump for one year and had to research and educate myself about lactation and pumping in order to pump long-term. It is my intention to provide you with the valuable information I have learned in order to help you make an informed decision about pumping. I also hope to enable you to both establish your supply and maintain your supply for, hopefully, as long as you would like to provide breast milk for your baby.

The information in this book is also based on the generosity of over 50 women who took the time to share with me the method by which they started to pump and how they maintained their supply. It is their experience which shows this is an option which is available to many.

It is difficult to argue that breast milk is not the best nutrition possible for our babies. When breastfeeding just doesn't work out, you can not breastfeed, or do not want to breastfeed but still recognize the value of breast milk, there is another option instead of formula. Women need to know this. You need to know this. While it is sometimes a more difficult road to travel, it is one that will be worth the effort when you look into the eyes of your breast milk-fed baby.

First Things First

When I had my son, I was surprised how emotional an experience it was. I was responsible for a new life, and it was the choices I made that would determine, to a large extent, my baby's health and physical and emotional development. I was also surprised by just how exhausting a venture it was to be a new mother, but I was determined to push through the difficulties and provide the very best for my child. Having a premature baby, with all the stress that naturally comes with it, and having a stressful, difficult experience trying to establish breastfeeding, I found myself at a crossroad: do I continue persevering and working to get him to breastfeed or do I make a choice to reduce the stress in our lives and move to bottle feed him exclusively?

Formula was never something I thought I would feed my child. It was just not an option I had ever considered, and yet when I encountered difficulty breastfeeding, suddenly I was facing this possibility. But I had been pumping since my son was born in order to establish my supply when he was too small to nurse, and I decided that this is what I would continue to do. I did not know if it was possible. I did not know if other women did it. I just knew that breast milk was the choice I wanted to make for my son and I would give it to him any way I could. So began my experience exclusively pumping.

I approach the subject of exclusively pumping with certain beliefs and biases:

1. Breastfeeding is the best way of nourishing a baby for at least the first year of life.

2. Breastfeeding does not always work out for numerous reasons.

3. When breastfeeding does not work out, breast milk is still the best way of nourishing a baby and it must then (in most cases) be provided by pumping.

4. Although many will say that pumping is breastfeeding, I consider it different. While the baby is receiving many of the benefits of breast milk, there are some benefits derived

from the act of breastfeeding which the baby will not receive. Therefore breastfeeding is superior in every respect.

5. Regardless of the method of delivery, breast milk is preferential to formula.

6. Breast milk for any length of time is better than no breast milk. Even if a woman decides to pump for a month or two or three, this is better for the baby than never benefiting from his mother's milk. A decision to pump does not have to be a year-long commitment.

7. All mothers make the choice that is best for their baby and best for their family. Women need to be supported in whatever choice they make, and they must be given the full spectrum of options available to them in order to make an informed decision.

8. Breastfeeding, and certainly exclusively pumping, is not always as encouraged and supported as it should be. Everyone surrounding a new mother should support breastfeeding and the option of exclusively pumping as an alternative to formula. It is important that those who work with new mothers have information about exclusively pumping and provide women with accurate information in order to support a woman considering the option.

9. Just as breastfeeding does not always work out for all women, not all women will find success exclusively pumping. Some women will not be able to pump enough milk, and some women will simply be overwhelmed by the time commitment necessary or the difficulty juggling a rigorous pumping schedule among all the many other aspects of life. A decision to use formula in order to supplement a low supply is sometimes necessary, and for some women, the effort of pumping will not seem worth it. This is an individual decision.

10. Although already stated, it is worth repeating a second time: breast milk, regardless of the delivery method is the best possible nutrition for a baby, and a mother must be encouraged and supported to provide breast milk for as long as she desires to do so. Mothers must have the option

of exclusively pumping presented to them if they do not want to breastfeed due to discomfort with the act itself or if breastfeeding does not work out for them.

Breast Milk Is Best For Baby

Methods of feeding have changed over the years. Today many healthy, intelligent adults can claim their start to being bottle fed formula. Over the past couple decades, breastfeeding has received the position it deserves, and now breast milk is rightfully seen as the optimal nutrition for infants. The World Health Organization recommends breastfeeding for at least the first year of a child's life. Most national pediatric associations recommend breastfeeding for six months as a minimum and often recommend a greater length of time. Large amounts of research money have been spent trying to fully understand the nutritional components of breast milk, and formula companies have continuously attempted to create a formula as closely resembling breast milk as possible. Of course an equivalent will never be created.

Mother's milk is remarkable in its ability to provide what a child needs and more remarkable in its ability to change as a child grows to provide the optimal nutrition for that stage of a child's life. The living aspect of breast milk makes it tremendously valuable for an infant's development and growth. The overall composition of breast milk is specifically designed for human infants, and formula will never match its quality.

Having said this, mother's make the choice that is best for their child, and sometimes this means feeding formula. It is the mother's right to choose. However, it is important that mothers are well informed, and more importantly, well supported when making their decision. Often a mother is so stressed over the feeding of a new baby that everyone begins to suffer. The pros and cons of formula feeding must be weighed. However, there is another option when a mother makes the decision to either stop breastfeeding or not to breastfeed at all: exclusively pumping.

Breast is Best

This mantra has taken the maternal world by storm. Every new and expecting mother has read it and been taught about it during pre-natal classes, in pregnancy and baby magazines and books, and from their doctors. The scientific data is unequivocal: breastfeeding is best for the child and for the mother. Breastfeeding not only provides optimal nutrition for the infant, it also provides long-term benefits for the mother.

Breastfeeding is by far the least complicated way to feed a baby. With no bottles to sterilize, no formula to prepare, and no bottles to warm, breastfeeding is practical and convenient for many. And perhaps one of the added benefits of breastfeeding is that mothers are able to enjoy a special bond with their baby and experience one-on-one time.

However, breastfeeding is not always possible and the "breast is best" cry often serves to make women who are not breastfeeding feel guilty. Often, mothers suffer immense emotional turmoil over the choice to stop breastfeeding- regardless of when this choice is made. Breastfeeding is supposed to be natural and womanly, and when it doesn't work out, feelings of guilt and inadequacy take over and sometimes lead women into depression. If the choice to stop breastfeeding or not breastfeed at all is due to complications in pregnancy, pain, or difficulty latching, a deep loss is often felt, and many women report going through a mourning period: mourning the loss of the relationship with their baby and the loss of the expectation they had to breastfeed. Many women are surprised at the strong emotions that well up when confronted with the possibility of no longer breastfeeding.

There are also women who choose not to breastfeed because they do not feel comfortable with the idea. Some of these women may have suffered sexual abuse and have difficulty disconnecting their breasts from the sexual abuse they experienced. Some have been raised in a family or culture where breastfeeding may have been considered primal and unenlightened. And some simply are not comfortable with the idea of a baby sucking at their breast. While it may be possible to overcome these issues with the help of a lactation consultant or other medical professional, no woman should be made to feel inadequate for her position and the decision should be left in her hands. Although, providing breastfeeding education to these mothers is of the utmost importance in order that they make their decision with all the facts in place.

Many, when making the decision to either stop breastfeeding or not to breastfeed at all, switch over to a cow's milk-based formula or soy-based formula. However, there is another option. This option is not as well known as the number of people choosing it might suggest. This option also often makes the decision to stop breastfeeding a little easier since it ensures that your baby can continue to receive breast milk. The option is to exclusively pump.

Breast Milk in Any Form is Better

Breastfeeding may be the most preferred method of feeding a baby, but it is the breast milk, after all, that is the main reason for this preference. By pumping breast milk and feeding it to your baby by bottle, your baby will receive many, although not all, of the benefits of breast milk that she would have received directly from the breast.

There has been little research completed on bottle feeding expressed breast milk, but it is logical to suggest that many of the benefits of breastfeeding are passed along through the breast milk itself. Of course, since breast milk is alive in its composition, the storage or freezing of expressed breast milk will naturally reduce its benefits. Yet when compared to the composition of formula, expressed breast milk is far superior.

Breastfeeding does provide some benefits that bottle feeding expressed breast milk will not such as proper oral development, convenience, and portability, but exclusively pumping should not be looked upon with disdain or puzzlement. Indeed, mothers who choose to exclusively pump should be lauded for their grand efforts. For not only are they bottle feeding, with all the additional work that is attached to it, but they are also producing the food that they are feeding and pumping sometimes eight to ten times a day to ensure their child gets the best they can provide. Most women who exclusively pump do not feel it was a decision they made but, instead, the only option left open to them.

The Importance of a Supportive Environment

Making the choice to exclusively pump requires support. Many well-meaning people have told women considering exclusively pumping that it is not a long-term option and that it is difficult to maintain your milk supply for an extended period with just a pump. While it is true that a baby is far better at establishing and maintaining a milk supply, the number of women who have been successful exclusively pumping suggest that it *is* possible and *is* an option. Some people even look upon the decision to exclusively pump negatively. They believe that it is a disservice to a baby and that every woman can breastfeed with enough dedication and effort. This attitude is one that forces some women to give up entirely and switch to formula, feeling inadequate for not being able to breastfeed.

The effects of stress and fatigue on a new mother are often overlooked or pushed aside in the attempts to establish a successful breastfeeding relationship. Sometimes, however, it is important to recognize that the mother needs to be healthy and functional in order to care for her child, and sometimes this will mean that the decision to stop breastfeeding may be a necessary one. Additional difficulties such as post-partum depression or family turmoil can, in and of themselves, create a difficult environment and the added stress of breastfeeding can become too much to handle.

Some people will also push the other way, stating that formulas are now excellent replacements for mother's milk and that the stress of trying to establish breastfeeding or exclusively pump is not worth it in the long run. While it is true that many babies do well on formula, there is still no formula that matches the exceptional qualities of breast milk.

In the end, the option to pump exclusively is often not provided at all to new or expecting mothers, but it is an option that needs to be shared. It is an option that people who work with new mothers must aware of in order to fully support women and babies.

When looking for support, look for a professional who is knowledgeable, supportive, and preferably someone who has had experience assisting other women through the process. Do not rely on advice that does not recognize exclusively pumping as being separate from breastfeeding in terms of maintaining and establishing supply as well as using a breast pump. While the goal is the same- to provide breast milk- the requirements to establish and maintain a supply exclusively with a pump are very different than simply pumping occasionally while breastfeeding.

Most importantly, find support! It can be a difficult road to travel, especially with a new baby at home. The first few weeks are tough and many women go through periods where quitting is on their minds constantly. But it is the knowledge that you are providing the best possible for your baby that will get you through. And as every woman who has exclusively pumped or is currently exclusively pumping will tell you, it gets easier! Seek out others who are pumping, whether they are in your community or on the Internet. The Internet is an excellent resource with many online discussion boards dedicated to those who are exclusively pumping due to varying circumstances (see "Resources").

Exclusively pumping can be a viable option when you get good information and the support you need! It can make it possible for a woman to provide her baby with the best nutrition possible: mother's milk.

The Reasons Women Exclusively Pump

The reasons for exclusively pumping are as varied as the women who exclusively pump. One thing all the women have in common, though, is their desire to provide breast milk for their babies. Whether the decision to exclusively pump is made by choice or desperation, due to an ill baby or the perceived loss of other options, the ability to exclusively pump allows women to feed expressed breast milk for longer than they would otherwise and allows them to forego the way of formula. Many women end up exclusively pumping when breastfeeding just doesn't work out for them; this can happen for a multitude of reasons. A large number of women also come to exclusively pump when their baby is born prematurely. For this group, pumping is a necessity if they wish to breastfeed, and, in some cases, breastfeeding can be very trying and difficult due to the many challenges a premature baby must overcome. And of course, prolonged illness and the separation of mother and baby can make breastfeeding impossible whereas pumping can allow the baby to still receive the goodness of breast milk.

Prematurity

Almost every women who delivers a premature baby before the thirty-fourth week of gestation must enter into the realm of pumping if she wishes to breastfeed her baby. Before the thirty-forth week of gestation, a baby simply does not have the strength or ability to latch and feed at the mother's breast. After thirty-four weeks (or thereabout), the baby can begin to attempt breastfeeding, but it may take a number of weeks before the baby is strong enough and has the required coordination to breastfeed well.

Pumping for the preemie is in many ways different than pumping for a full-term baby. With a premature infant, the hope is usually that the baby will eventually be able to be put to breast and indeed breastfeed exclusively. While this is a possibility, and many women are successful at getting their preemies to breastfeed, there are also many women who are not able to breastfeed their preemie for a variety of reasons. Often, the mother will feel that providing breast milk for her baby is about the only thing that she can do for her baby while he is in the hospital. Pumping becomes her full-time job and her most important mission at that moment in time.

Pumping for the premature infant is extremely important since it is the pumping that will establish the milk supply and provide a good foundation for long-term milk production. In other situations, it is the baby that establishes supply through frequent nursing, but with a preemie, it is the pumping that must be frequent. Frustration and exhaustion are part of the norm for mothers, and with the stress of having a premature baby on top of the exhausting pumping schedule, it is easy to become overwhelmed.

Mothers need to be sure they take care of themselves: sleep when they can, eat well, and ensure they are drinking enough water. It is easy to lose sight of the big picture and forget why you are pumping. A baby needs his mother: a mother who is healthy and strong. Becoming consumed with pumping and calculating total daily volumes can easily take over your life. While breast milk is extremely valuable for a premature baby and will provide the optimum nutrition, more important is a mother who is able to be there for her child. Balance your life and your efforts. Consider carefully the options and do not be afraid to admit it is too much for you. Ask for help- demand help- and accept help when it is offered.

In the case of a preemie, a hospital-grade pump is your best option. Since you do not have the benefit of nursing to establish your supply, use the best quality pump available to ensure success down the road. Once established, you may choose to change to a personal pump, but now is not the time to skimp or experiment. Mothers of preemies, especially very early preemies, may have a more difficult time establishing their supply since their breasts might not have fully prepared for milk production before the birth of their baby and their hormone levels might not be adequate. It is important to be aware of this, adopt good pumping habits, and seek out the advice of a lactation consultant who has experience working with mothers of premature babies.

Pumping for the preemie also has the added requirement of transporting your breast milk to the hospital. The Infant Intensive Care Unit should provide you with their guidelines for handling breast milk for a preemie. Be sure to follow them carefully. It is important to remember that the premature baby is more fragile than a full-term baby and it is vital that breast milk be handled with the utmost care to ensure it is free from contaminants and stored as safely as possible.

Latch Problems

While breastfeeding is a natural thing, it does not always come naturally. Women and babies need to learn how to breastfeed. Occasionally, a baby may develop problems with her latch which makes it difficult to continue to breastfeed. Problems include a baby who will not latch, a shallow latch, a sleepy baby, cleft palate, and painful latch. While it may be possible to correct many of these problems, the baby's health and a lack of weight gain can become an issue. Of primary importance is the health of the baby, and if the baby is not eating well, then chances are they are also not gaining weight well and might even become dehydrated. The mother's primary concern is the health of her baby, so bottle feeding often becomes the method of feeding in order to ensure the baby is able to eat satisfactory volumes. At this point, the mother must decide what will be in the bottle.

Although there are other methods of feeding a baby instead of using a bottle and nipple (such as a Supplemental Nursing System (SNS), finger feeding, or cup feeding), bottle feeding is usually the most common method used when a baby needs to be supplemented or fed in an alternate way. It is, of course, possible to turn to bottle feeding for a short period while you continue to work on the latch. Just because a baby has been given a bottle does not mean they will never breastfeed. However, it is possible for a baby to develop a preference for the bottle nipple since the flow is often faster and the baby does not have to work as hard to receive the milk. It is possible to get a baby back to breast even if they are two or three months old. Sometimes a baby just needs to get stronger in order for things to work out.

So if you are unable to breastfeed from the beginning, but really want to, don't give up.

Sometimes, women who exclusively pump will continue to breastfeed their child simply for comfort as opposed to nourishment. This often will allow for the special bonding and closeness of breastfeeding even though the bottle is still used for feeding. This ability to still breastfeed in a limited manner can ease the feelings of loss over not being able to breastfeed exclusively. In these situations, the baby is often able to latch but will not nurse long enough to take a full feed or perhaps has become accustomed to bottle feeding and no longer nurses when hungry.

If you have latching problems with your baby, it is extremely important to seek out the advice of an expert in the field of lactation. A lactation consultant will observe a breastfeeding session, diagnose problems, and can provide excellent advice on how to solve these problems. With the right strategies in place, many problems can be overcome and a happy, successful breastfeeding relationship established. However, if you decide that you can no longer breastfeed, exclusively pumping is a viable alternative to formula.

Illness

Illness, of the mother or the baby, can lead a woman to exclusively pumping. Anything that limits the contact of mother and baby will put a successful breastfeeding relationship at risk. A baby that is too ill to nurse will require alternative feeding methods and may be able to be fed breast milk by either bottle or NG tube.

The illness of the mother makes the possibility of exclusively pumping more difficult, but, depending on circumstances, it may be possible. As with any other reason to exclusively pump, all the options must be weighed and a realistic look at the requirements must be taken. Depending on the mother's illness, exclusively pumping may not be possible due to the strict schedule required at the outset or medications that the mother is taking; however, it is worth discussing this option with medical professionals including a lactation consultant and your medical doctors. Ultimately, the decision will be made by you in consultation with the medical community.

The illness of a baby may create a number of reasons that breastfeeding would not be possible: hospitalization, lack of strength, or inability to eat orally resulting in the requirement of a tube for feeding. In all these situations, many mothers desire to provide the absolute best for their child, and, once again, breast milk is the best nutrition possible. Pumping for an ill child can be extremely taxing on a mother who has many additional stresses in her life due to the illness of her child. But on the other hand, exclusively pumping for that child can provide the mother with a sense of empowerment, allowing her to nurture her child in this special way.

Separation

When mother and baby are separated for long periods, breastfeeding, of course, becomes extremely difficult. By pumping, the mother can provide breast milk for her baby even though she can not be with the child. Nursing can continue when possible, and by pumping, the mother can maintain her supply.

Separation from your baby will require careful attention to the collection, storage, and transportation of the expressed breast milk. Depending on the distance you need to travel, this may be more challenging, but it is possible. Verse yourself in the safe storage and handling of expressed breast milk and determine the best possible methods for your particular situation. Contacting your local health unit for information on safe food handling is an excellent first step.

Choice

Some women turn to exclusively pumping by choice. They have determined prior to giving birth that they do not want to breastfeed, but they are convinced that the best nutrition for their child is breast milk. The reasons for this choice are varied. Some women simply do not like the idea of a baby sucking at their breast. Other women may have been sexually abused and have difficulty separating the abuse from their bodies. And some women may feel that exclusively pumping will provide them will more freedom than breastfeeding would. Regardless of the reason, the choice to exclusively pump will provide a superior option over commercially prepared formulas.

If you decide to pump from the beginning without attempting to breastfeed, be sure your doctor and the hospital staff are aware of your wishes. Ensure that your spouse or the person who will be with you during labour and delivery are comfortable in standing up for your choice and willing to make your wishes known to the staff. Research the availability of breast pumps in the delivery ward, and, if necessary, bring your own pump with you. You may need to have your own pump cleared through the hospital building/electrical staff before using it, so find this out ahead of time.

Regardless of the reasons for exclusively pumping, the most important thing is to get support and knowledge. It is vitally important to initiate a strong supply in order to see long-term success.

The Decision to Exclusively Pump

Before committing yourself to the idea of exclusively pumping, it is important to be completely prepared for the ups and downs of this decision. There are many emotions that you may have surrounding the issue of breastfeeding: some internally based and some may originate externally. Be prepared for these emotions to surface if you decide to exclusively pump. It is also important to have a realistic picture of what you are getting involved in. For some women, the ability to feed breast milk will far outweigh any negatives attached to exclusively pumping. However, most women, at some point in time, will find the daily requirements taxing and reconsider their decision. It is important to have the support of family and friends behind you. Exclusively pumping takes up more time than other options and can impact the daily lives of your loved ones. As well, be sure you are familiar with all of your options before you commit to exclusively pumping. By being as well informed as possible, you can ensure as high a likelihood of success as possible.

Emotions

As if being a mother wasn't emotional enough! Having to make a decision about how to feed your child when breastfeeding is no longer an option can bring to the surface many strong emotions. If breastfeeding was something you really wanted to do and something you looked upon as a bonding experience with your baby, the loss of this relationship may hit you very hard.

Many moms report going through a grieving period when they are no longer able to breastfeed. However, the opportunity to continue feeding your baby breast milk can help to ease this sense of loss. These feelings often centre on inadequacy and a feeling of failure. In fact, many women, when discussing their switch to exclusively pumping, will state that breastfeeding was a "failure" or they "failed" at breastfeeding. It often takes time to overcome these emotions and talking to other women about your experience can be a great help.

It is important to remember that you need to take care of yourself in order to take care of your baby. While in the middle of making the decision to stop breastfeeding, many women are completely overwhelmed. They are extremely sleep deprived, possibly in pain due to thrush or a poor latch, frustrated, and feeling inadequate. These feelings only serve to increase the stress that new moms are feeling.

Seeking out the support and advice of professionals such as doctors or lactation consultants can be extremely helpful, but be prepared for it to possibly put more pressure on you to either continue to breastfeed, persevere through the problems you are facing, or else to switch to formula. Sometimes people think about the good of the baby but forget about the good of the mother. While breastfeeding can be good for both, the stress and strain of trying to establish breastfeeding can quickly take its toll and leave you with nothing left to give your baby.

Weigh your options carefully and objectively.

Ask yourself these questions:

- How long can you continue as you are now?
- How much support do you have to continue to breastfeed?
- How much support do you have if you decide to exclusively pump?
- Have there been other extenuating circumstances surrounding the birth of your baby that have added to the stress you are feeling (e.g. illness, prematurity, c-section)?
- How will you feel in a few months about your decision if you stop breastfeeding?
- Are there any other avenues of support that you can use?
- Is your baby thriving?
- Are you constantly concerned about your baby's well-being and her ability to take adequate feeds?

While it is possible to get your baby back to breast if you stop breastfeeding for a while, it is more likely that you will not return to exclusive breastfeeding, so you need to be comfortable with your decision and prepared for the emotions that you will feel as a result of it.

You will be confronted by people who do not understand your decision to exclusively pump. People will tell you that it is impossible. Some may say that you are doing your baby a disservice by not breastfeeding. And yet others will tell you that you might as well switch to formula since it would be easier. There will always be someone who will question your decision, but in the end it is you who needs to be comfortable with it.

On the other hand, you will meet people who will respect and admire your determination and commitment to exclusively pump for your baby. These are the people you want to keep close!

Almost every mother I have talked to admits to having feelings of guilt and loss over not breastfeeding. Breastfeeding is our womanly right; it is what we do. Other possibilities are often not even considered until the day you are confronted by the fact that breastfeeding is not working out as you had expected. Coming to terms with not breastfeeding can take time. Taking it as a personal failure is a natural response but one that is not helpful in any way. Focus on the facts and on the positives:

- A mother trying to cope under an increasing burden of stress is eventually going to break, whether it be her emotional or physical well-being that suffers.
- A baby needs his mother.
- The maternal bond is much more than the method of feeding.
- Even though you are not breastfeeding directly, your baby is still benefiting from your breast milk.
- Mothering is filled with guilt- this won't be the first thing for which you feel guilt!
- It is often possible to continue to breastfeed for comfort if not return to breastfeeding exclusively.
- Once you see how well your baby does receiving your breast milk, your decision will be much easier to accept.
- And if nothing else, the fact that you exclusively pumped, with all the hard work and time that goes into it, will be a wonderful thing to tell your child about

when he is giving you grief in his teenage years: "When you were a baby, I loved you so much, that I…".

The Realities of Exclusively Pumping

Depending on when you talk to a mother who is exclusively pumping, she will tell you it's the hardest thing she has ever done or that it is simply part of her daily routine and can allow for some added freedom in her life due to the fact that others can feed the baby. The truth of exclusively pumping is that it can be a roller coaster of emotions, but, as every mother will also tell you, it gets easier.

The irony of switching to exclusively pumping from breastfeeding is that you usually make the switch because you are completely overwhelmed trying to establish breastfeeding or you are having difficulties such as painful thrush or a poor latch. The decision to switch to exclusively pumping will not necessarily remove the feeling of being overwhelmed, but it can allow you to see a light at the end and allow you to refocus on solving any lingering problems. Having to pump frequently, and around the clock, can be extremely tiring and exhausting. Pain caused by a yeast infection will not go away because you decide to pump, and you will now need to worry about sterilizing everything you use to pump in order to get rid of the yeast. A painful latch will not necessarily transfer over to a problem with the pump, but if your nipples have been traumatized, they may be sensitive to the pump as well.

However, most women find that exclusively pumping is an option that is possible long-term. They no longer see their baby unhappy and frustrated at breast; they are completely aware of how much their babies are eating and are able to see them thrive; since others can help in the feeding of the baby, it is possible (although not always practical) that mom can get some extra sleep; and since baby is still receiving mother's milk and not formula, mom feels good about the nutrition that baby is receiving.

Once you get into the routine of pumping, it becomes just that- routine. However, exclusively pumping is more work than either breastfeeding or formula feeding. In fact, in many ways it is doing both of the other options together. Be aware of this before you start. Not only does it take time to pump (usually about two hours a day of pumping) but it also takes time to clean and sterilize bottles and pumping equipment as well as time to bottle feed your baby. Once again, it comes down to your reasons for exclusively pumping. How important is it to you for your baby to receive breast milk? For those women who have chosen to exclusively pump, it is well worth the extra time and energy.

When you initially start to exclusively pump, the time requirement will be much greater than a few months in. It is important to pump frequently when you are first establishing your supply. Once your supply becomes established, you will be able to drop pumping sessions-slowly! However, as you drop sessions you will usually need to increase the length of time you are pumping, so in general, you will pump for the same total time each day. Although, since you are not pumping as often, you will gain some freedom from the pump and be able to fit pumping into your daily schedule instead of fitting your daily schedule into your pumping routine. The cautious time to start dropping pumps is around three months post-partum; yet, many women have started dropping sessions earlier than this with no ill effect. The most common reason women give for dropping a session is the inability to keep up the pace they were going and the need for the extra time in their life.

The extra work and time commitment involved with exclusively pumping usually diminish as you go along. Whether you just get used to the schedule or completely forget what it would be like with the extra time in your life, it does get easier.

The two things that don't necessarily get easier, though, and things that you will personally need to deal with, are your feelings towards no longer breastfeeding and the possible lack of support for your decision to exclusively pump from those around you. However, in many ways women who are exclusively pumping are breastfeeding; the delivery method is just a little different. And I can't think of a stronger breastfeeding advocate than a mother who is willing to hook up to a breast pump eight or more times a day to ensure her baby is able to receive breast milk.

What to Expect

There are a number of things that almost every woman who exclusively pumps can expect at some point on her journey. Here they are, both the positives and the negatives:

The Positives

- Looking into the eyes of your breast milk-fed baby and knowing that everything you are doing will benefit your baby for years to come

If the first positive is not enough:

- Expect to pay far less than you would if you were feeding formula
- Feelings of pride and accomplishment
- Many people will respect your dedication and effort to feed your baby breast milk
- Ability to have others feed the baby
- Multiple health and cognitive benefits from feeding breast milk
- Health benefits for the mother due to lactation

The Negatives

- Lack of sleep (not that this is exclusive to moms who pump, but the pumping will take more time away from sleep)
- Sore nipples and breast pain (this doesn't have to be a foregone conclusion, but be prepared for it because it often does happen although it is often because of improper equipment or pumping techniques)
- Misinformed people and people who want to know why you are not breastfeeding
- Feelings of resentment towards your pump (in the early weeks and months many women feel "attached" to their pump- physically, not emotionally- but this will pass)

- Difficulty juggling a baby and a rigorous pumping schedule (there must be some law about babies that when the pump turns on, baby screams)
- Overwhelming desires to quit (everyone has been here- you are not alone)

For information and ideas on how to overcome the difficulties sometimes associated with exclusively pumping, see the chapter "Overcoming Difficulties".

Know Your Options

Most people, if asked, would state that there are two options to feed a baby: breastfeeding and formula feeding. There is, of course, the third option to exclusively pump. It is important that you understand all of your options before making the decision to exclusively pump and to go into the decision with as much knowledge as possible.

If you are currently breastfeeding, but thinking about exclusively pumping, consider the options you have before you:

- You can continue to breastfeed.
- You can switch to formula.
- You can seek professional help from a lactation consultant to assist you in establishing a successful breastfeeding relationship if you are currently having difficulties.

As previously mentioned, exclusively pumping is demanding and a lot of work. For most women, breastfeeding will be less effort and often will be the best thing for both mother and baby. If you are considering exclusively pumping because you think it will be easier, less work, or allow you more time for yourself, please reconsider. Not only is this not the case for most women, but your baby will be missing some of the benefits of direct breastfeeding. If you do not want to continue breastfeeding full-time, consider pumping in addition to breastfeeding. This will allow you some freedom to go out, work, or sleep and have your partner feed the baby, but will also allow you the flexibility to breastfeed when necessary, provide you with the closeness derived from breastfeeding, and continue to provide your baby with some of the benefits of direct breastfeeding.

For those women who are having difficulty establishing breastfeeding for whatever reason, the ability to pump can allow you to maintain your supply until you can solve whatever is causing the difficulty. Consider getting advice and assistance from a lactation consultant. Your local hospital or health unit should be able to connect you with someone who can meet with you and your baby and troubleshoot the situation. You may also find private practice lactation consultants listed in the Yellow Pages under "Breastfeeding" or "Lactation". While not every problem can be solved, nor is everyone able to last under the stress of the situation, it is a good idea to work with a lactation consultant. Direct breastfeeding is the best choice when possible, and it is worth seeking assistance before choosing another road.

And of course, for every situation, the other alternative is to feed commercially prepared formula. While some will say that it is an acceptable alternative, the honest statement is that it is the best alternative if breast milk is not available. Breast milk is by far the best nutrition for infants. Commercial formulas will never come close. Breast milk is living. It is able to change to meet the needs of your baby. It passes immunity to your child. It is the easiest for a baby to digest and provides the exact building blocks that an infant requires, not just for his current needs, but for his future needs as well.

Having said that, the success of formula companies today tells us that people are feeding their infants formula. It is a fact that breastfeeding is not something that every mother will choose. If you are faced with this decision, you owe it to your baby to be well informed. Gather as much information as you can about breast milk and formula. Learn for yourself what the benefits are and make an educated decision. Most moms who choose to exclusively pump do so because they believe that breast milk is the best food for their baby, and they are willing to go the extra mile to provide it.

Feelings of Guilt

Often women who decide to exclusively pump (and mothers who formula feed) express feelings of guilt over their decision not to breastfeed or their inability to breastfeed. If you wanted to breastfeed but were unable to do so, you may need to work through your emotions surrounding the loss of this special relationship with your baby. Some women also struggle with the belief that they gave in too easily and did not try hard enough to successfully breastfeed.

In most cases, these feelings of guilt arise because of a strong desire to breastfeed. You had certain expectations before the birth of your child, and suddenly those expectations are not coming to fruition. You find yourself pumping breast milk or feeding formula and it isn't what you wanted or planned. It isn't the choice you would make given the option, and you may feel like things are happening to you instead of you having control over what is happening.

In order to reduce the feelings of guilt you may have, it is important to do everything you can to make the breastfeeding relationship with your baby possible, if this is what you want. In your mind, ensure that you have done everything you were able to do. The "what ifs" that can haunt you otherwise can make what is already an emotional time even more difficult.

Understand the options you do have in front of you. We rarely in life have no choice in what we do. If you consciously make the choice to exclusively pump or feed formula you will feel more in control than if you just let the choice happen. Decide what you want to do after carefully considering your options and make the decision based on the needs of your family.

If you are feeling extreme guilt or sadness, or if you have any negative thoughts towards your baby, seek out the assistance of a physician. Post-partum depression can be very serious, and with the added stress of breastfeeding difficulties, an ill or premature baby, or your own illness or recovery after surgery, depression can be even more apt to occur. Take care of your own health so you can take care of your baby.

Generally, the strong emotions women who are exclusively pumping experience can be more accurately labeled as grief, disappointment, anger, and sadness. Often though, it is described as guilt.

Making Your Decision

Now that you know the reality of exclusively pumping- the negative aspects as well as the positive ones- you will need to decide. The decision is yours to make. Trust your instincts. Don't allow yourself to feel guilty about making the decision. Don't allow others to force their will upon you. You are your baby's mother, and your baby needs you. You need to make the decision that will be right for both of you. This decision is different for every woman, and it is made for different reasons. You may perhaps continue to breastfeed. You may decide to switch to formula. You may decide to exclusively pump. Whatever decision you do make, be sure you are making it for the right reasons. The decision will feel right and allow you to enjoy your baby knowing that you are doing what is right for her.

Breast Milk:
The Production, Composition, and Benefits

In order to successfully pump long-term, it is necessary to have a basic understanding of lactation and the composition of breast milk. While it is not essential to have a deep, scientific knowledge, it is beneficial to have a general sense of how things happen in order to make informed decisions about your pumping schedule. There are many books already published that go into great detail about the structures of the breast and the process of lactation. I would encourage you to search out these books at your local library. This chapter will deal with the information that is particularly relevant to those women who are exclusively pumping.

Lactation

During pregnancy, the glandular tissue of the breasts grows and replaces the fatty tissue. As early as sixteen weeks gestation, a woman's breasts will begin to produce colostrum. However, it is not until the third trimester that milk producing cells completely mature. Mothers of premature babies under thirty-two weeks gestation, especially first time mothers, may have difficulty initiating a strong supply due to the fact that their breasts have not developed sufficiently to produce milk.

Lactogenesis (or the beginning of breast milk production) occurs in three distinct stages:

Stage one begins in the weeks prior to a full-term delivery. There is an increase seen in the elements needed for breast milk production: lactose, total protein, immunoglobulins.

Stage two begins immediately after delivery of the placenta. The removal of the placenta marks a sharp decrease in the level of pregnancy hormones within the mother. This stage continues in the days following delivery up to when a woman's milk "comes in". During this stage there is increased blood flow to the breasts as well as increased oxygen, glucose, and citrate. This stage will happen regardless of whether a woman chooses to breastfeed or not and regardless of whether a baby, or pump, stimulates the breast.

Stage three is the establishment of a mature milk supply.

The production of breast milk is dynamic and active. The breast responds to the stimulation of an infant with a series of events that release hormones, which in turn stimulate a milk ejection reflex, or let-down, and prompt further production or signal to decrease production if, for some reason, the milk is not removed from the breast. Once stage two lactogenesis has begun, milk production is largely controlled by the baby, or in the case of a woman exclusively pumping, controlled by the pump and frequency of pumping sessions.

Three things are necessary to maintain breast milk supply:

- there must be the required hormones present and they must successfully travel to the breast (known as endocrine control);
- there must be stimulation to the nipple, areola, and breast;
- and the milk within the breast must be removed (known as autocrine control).

It has also been shown that the fuller the breast, the slower milk production becomes. Frequent removal of milk is important and, if trying to build a supply, frequency is critical.

Two Key Hormones in Breast Milk Production

Prolactin

Prolactin, a hormone, is produced in the anterior pituitary gland. It is essential for the complete development of the breast during pregnancy. After the delivery of the placenta and the dramatic decrease of pregnancy hormones, prolactin levels initiate the milk supply. Prolactin is released in waves, and its levels are directly related to the stimulation of the areola, nipple, and breast.

One recent theory about breast milk production is the theory of prolactin receptors. Prolactin receptors, which are proteins found on the surface of cells and that bind to prolactin triggering breast cells to utilize the hormone, are established during the first few weeks post-partum. Frequent stimulation of the nipple, areolas, and breasts will increase the number of prolactin receptors in the breast. Frequent pumping, or breastfeeding, is essential to developing a strong milk supply, and the prolactin receptor theory suggests why this is so. In many ways, prolactin receptors are more important than prolactin levels, since without the receptors, the simple presence of prolactin will do very little. Also, when prolactin levels naturally start to drop off several weeks post-partum, it is the prolactin receptors that will make the most of the reduced prolactin levels and assist in maintaining a strong supply. However, once the endocrine control of breast milk production diminishes, it is the autocrine control which becomes primary: milk removal means more milk produced.

Prolactin levels peak during the night, and therefore pumping at night will assist in building your milk supply and make the most of those high levels. It is recommended by many pumping moms that you pump at least once during the night between the hours of 1 a.m. and 5 a.m. for the first three months post-partum or at least until your baby starts sleeping through the night.

Prolactin also inhibits the maturing and release of eggs from the ovaries. The absence of menstruation during lactation is known as lactational amenorrhea. This highlights just another reason why frequent pumping to increase your level of prolactin is beneficial.

It is important to note that progesterone may interfere with normal prolactin production and its interaction with cell receptors. Progestin-only birth control is the best oral contraceptive to use while lactating, however, due to the possibility that it may interfere with the establishment of the milk supply, it is usually recommended that you wait until your supply is well established before starting progestin-only birth control. Oral contraceptives containing estrogen are not recommended for lactating women. Seek the advice of a knowledgeable physician who is experienced with lactation and the possible effects of birth control. If you do take hormonal birth control and find that your supply is starting to decline, stop immediately and use a different form of birth control.

Oxytocin

Oxytocin is a hormone connected to the milk ejection reflex (MER). Oxytocin receptors in the breast increase during pregnancy and also increase in the uterus prior to delivery. The uterus uses oxytocin to prevent post-partum hemorrhages by contracting the uterus. Oxytocin is released from the pituitary gland when the nipple is stimulated.

Oxytocin acts upon the smooth muscles of the breast and causes contractions which push the milk into the ducts and to the nipple. The MER, or let-down, takes place multiple times during a feeding or pumping session since the oxytocin is released in waves as stimulation continues. As a new wave of oxytocin is released, a new MER will occur. This knowledge is important for the mother who is exclusively pumping. Many women will stop pumping once their milk flow has stopped having been told they should pump only a few minutes after the flow of milk has stopped. However, since the MER is initiated by waves of oxytocin being released, the flow of milk will also come in waves. It may take two or more let-downs in order to remove a sufficient amount of milk from your breasts. The autocrine system of control (milk removed = more milk produced) takes over from the hormonally maintained system of early milk production. You must remove the milk from your breasts in order to maintain your supply, and this means understanding that the MER is not continuous but occurs intermittently.

Stages of Breast Milk

There are three stages of breast milk:

Colostrum is the first milk to be produced. It is yellow to orange in colour and is very thick and somewhat sticky. Colostrum works as a laxative for a newborn assisting them in ridding their body of meconium. If meconium is not removed from a baby's system, it can lead to jaundice since their body will reabsorb the bilirubin from the meconium.

If pumping, it is important to collect and feed colostrum, not only for the laxative effect, but because it is highly concentrated with valuable immunity which will assist your baby in fighting off infections. While some mothers choose to supplement with formula at birth, this is not necessary and is perhaps not the best thing for the baby. Colostrum will assist the baby's digestive system to begin its work and not force it to work full-force immediately at birth.

Transitional milk follows colostrum. It can be seen as early as twelve hours after delivery and usually lasts one to two weeks. It is the consistency of mature milk, but it retains some of the colour of colostrum.

Mature milk has a slight bluish tinge to it and is rather thin when compared to formula or whole cow's milk. It contains all the nutrition that a baby needs for at least the first six months of life. Breast milk will continue to change throughout lactation, responding to the needs of the infant, the mother's exsposure to virus and bacteria, and the mother's diet.

Composition of Breast Milk

Breast milk is an amazing combination of fats, proteins, vitamins, minerals, growth factors, hormones, enzymes, and immuno-protective elements. Even when a mother is not receiving adequate nutrition, she will still be able to provide the necessary nutrients to her baby. Lactation will occur regardless of a mother's nutritional status.

While lactation will occur regardless of whether the mother is eating a well-balanced diet, the levels of certain elements in breast milk are determined by the mother's intake while other elements are not. Carbohydrate and protein levels are not greatly affected by the mother's food consumption and tend to remain at a relatively constant level. However, the level of fats in breast milk can vary depending on a number of factors. Vitamin and mineral levels are also related to the mother's own intake.

The greater bioactivity (meaning the ability for it to affect living cells) and bioavailability (meaning it is more easily absorbed and used) of breast milk make it far superior to formula even when levels of certain elements are low. While a lactating woman should of course make every effort to eat as nutritiously as possible, poor diet should not be a reason not to provide breast milk.

The volume of milk a mother produces is not greatly affected by her diet. Milk production remains at a fairly constant level. In addition, increasing your intake of fluids will not increase your volume of milk. It is important to remain well hydrated; however, it is not necessary to drink excessive amounts of water or other fluids.

Specific elements found in breast milk:

Proteins

- proteins are not affected by the nutrition of the mother
- provide the baby with immune and non-immune protection

Fat

- fats are greatly impacted by the nutrition of the mother
- also affected by length of gestation, length of lactation, number of children mother has had, and weight changes of the mother
- mothers of premature babies will produce milk that has a higher fat content and it will stay at higher levels for the first few months of lactation
- weight gain during pregnancy has a direct correlation to a higher fat content in breast milk
- fat content increases as the breast empties
- the higher the volume of milk you are producing, the lower the amount of fat in that milk

Vitamins and Minerals

- vitamin and mineral levels depend on the mother's own vitamin and mineral status
- vitamin D should be supplemented if daily sunlight exposure is limited
- iron in breast milk is highly bioavailable, meaning even small amounts of iron are more readily absorbed than the larger amounts found in formula
- breast milk contains an element, lactoferrin, that binds with iron making it easier for the baby to utilize

Immune and Non-immune Protecting Properties

- the production of these protective elements relate closely to the baby's own ability to produce their own immunity
- as the baby's own immune system begins to work independently, the protective properties of breast milk start to decrease
- during the baby's gestation, and during her first few months of life, the mother provides passive immunity to the baby (transfers immunity through the blood stream and then through breast milk)
- passive immunity is extremely effective for the first six months of a baby's life. After this time, the space between the cells of the baby's small intestine "closes" making it more difficult for the relatively large antibodies and other proteins to pass through into the baby's blood stream.
- the immune properties of breast milk have been shown to reduce incidence of necrotizing enterocolitis, diarrhea, respiratory infections, otitis media, diabetes, lymphoma, Crohn's disease, and urinary tract infections
- also contains antiviral, antiprotozoan, and antibacterial properties
- increased immune function in breast milk-fed babies can be seen not only when they are receiving the milk, but for several years after weaning
- it also may be that the immune systems of breast milk-fed babies mature more rapidly than their formula-fed counterparts

Growth Factors and Hormones

- growth factors and hormones are essential for proper growth and development
- stimulate the production of blood cells and the maintenance and repair of tissue

Enzymes

- assist baby with functions that have not yet fully developed such as pancreatic functions and digestive functions

Benefits of Breast Milk

Breast milk is amazing in its ability to provide not just adequate nutrition, but superior nutrition as well as protective and long-lasting benefits. But not only is breast milk valuable to babies, lactation itself is proving to provide numerous health and psychological benefits to mothers.

While most research on the benefits of breast milk investigate those babies who are breastfeeding, it is possible, in many instances, to transfer this understanding of breast milk to the breast milk-fed baby. However, not all benefits of breastfeeding are found in the breast milk itself. And while all mothers strive to create a strong, personal bond with their child, it is more difficult to achieve the same type of contact a breastfeeding mother and baby enjoy.

It is important when considering whether or not to exclusively pump to recognize that there are some benefits of breastfeeding that your child will not receive. If you are able to breastfeed, then that option will allow your baby to receive the entire range of benefits. However, the majority of benefits are found in the breast milk itself and breast milk feeding remains a far superior choice when compared to commercially prepared formulas.

The following tables provide a list of benefits to both baby and mother that will be received through breast milk and lactation as well as a comparison of direct breastfeeding and breast milk feeding.

It is important to note that the benefits of breast milk feeding are optimal with freshly pumped breast milk and that some properties may be reduced or destroyed by storage.

Benefits of Breast Milk for Baby: Comparison of Benefits from Direct Breastfeeding and Breast Milk Feeding

Benefit to Baby	Breastfeeding	Breast Milk Feeding
Colostrum acts as a laxative to help clear meconium out of baby's system and reduce incidence of jaundice	●	●
Provides immunity to baby and helps baby's own immune system mature	●	●
Lowers risks of ear infections, pneumonias, gastroenteritis, botulism, bacterial meningitis	●	●
Provides protection from chronic diseases such as lymphoma, Crohn's, celiac disease, ulcerative colitis, juvenile rheumatoid arthritis, insulin dependent diabetes	●	●
Baby will have a better response to childhood immunizations	●	●
Reduction in allergies, asthma, and eczema	●	●
Reduced risk of obesity	●	? *
Optimal brain development	●	●
Higher I.Q. scores than formula-fed counterparts	●	●
Reduces risk of necrotizing enterocolitis, especially important in premature babies	●	●
Protects from viral, bacterial, and parasitic infection	●	●
Benefits are long-lasting; remain after weaning from breast milk	●	●
Optimal oral development	●	
Possibly reduces the risk of Sudden Infant Death Syndrome	●	?**
Lowers risk of tooth decay caused by baby bottle	●	
Increases hand-eye coordination	●	
Close skin-to-skin contact enhances mother-child bonding	●	?***

Benefits of Lactation for the Mother: Comparison of Benefits from Direct Breastfeeding and Breast Milk Feeding

Benefit to Mother	Breastfeeding	Breast Milk Feeding
Healthy baby while receiving breast milk and healthier baby long-term	●	●
Waves of oxytocin post-partum help to return uterus to pre-pregnancy size and decrease the risk of hemorrhages after delivery	●	●
Delayed return of ovulation and period	●	●
Decreased risk of iron deficiency due to lactational amenorrhea	●	●
May cause easier weight loss post-partum, but not for all women	●	●
Decreases the risk of breast cancer, ovarian cancer, and uterine cancer	●	●
May reduce the risk of developing osteoporosis	●	●
Hormones produced during lactation may help to establish a closer bond with baby	●	●
Skin-to-skin contact creates close bond	●	?***

* The effects of breastfeeding on obesity are still disputed. If it does play a role in maintaining a future healthy weight, it is unknown what causes the correlation. One possibility is that breastfeeding allows a baby to self-regulate their eating whereas bottle feeding (regardless of what is in the bottle) tends to allow a baby to eat more and parents often encourage a baby to finish the entire bottle. The other possibility is that the components of breast milk themselves play a role in decreasing the likelihood of obesity later in life.

** The relationship between Sudden Infant Death Syndrome (SIDS) and breastfeeding is not entirely clear. There have been studies that show a small positive correlation between the two. However, other risk-reduction measures such as laying the baby on his back to sleep, removing any fluffy bedding from the crib, and parents not smoking are, in combination, a greater benefit. If breastfeeding does decrease the risk of SIDS, the cause is unclear. It is possible that the close contact between a mother and breastfed baby may impact the risks. It is also a possibility that the reduced number of infections in a breastfed baby lower the risk of SIDS. In the latter case, breast milk-fed babies would also see the benefit.

*** The benefits of skin-to-skin contact are entirely dependent on whether a mother chooses to do this with her baby. Skin-to-skin contact is not a benefit solely for breastfeeding though and can be experienced with a bottle fed baby as well.

The Fundamentals of Exclusively Pumping

How to Pump

Beyond the actual placing of the pump flanges to your breasts and turning on the pump, there are some useful guidelines and suggestions that will make your experience more productive and less tedious.

- Double pump! Not only will double pumping save you time, you will also make the most of your prolactin levels by double pumping. Be sure the pump you decide on has the capability to double pump.

- Ensure your nipples are centred in the flanges. If not, this can cause excessive friction and soreness.

- Enjoy lots of skin-to-skin contact with your baby, especially early on. Not only is this a nice, restful and intimate time to share with your new baby, it will encourage your milk production. Many mothers find that they will pump more milk after snuggling with their baby.

- Think of your baby while you are pumping. Attach a photograph to your pump. Watch your baby sleeping. Think of her smile. This will assist you in letting down for the pump and help you to relax.

- Buy extra pump kits and have lots of collection bottles. This way you will not have to wash your kit after every pump. You can do the cleaning once or twice a day. Many kits can be washed in the dishwasher as well.

- Buy a steam sterilizer. If you do not have a dishwasher that will wash at a high enough temperature to sterilize, consider buying a steam sterilizer. It will save you a lot of time and ensure your pump kit, as well as your collection and feeding bottles, are sterilized.

- Use lanolin to prevent excess friction. While this is not an absolute necessity, many mothers find the use of lanolin beneficial in reducing any possible chafing and it will help keep your nipples soft. Do not use lanolin if you have thrush. Some mothers choose to use olive oil instead of lanolin. Olive oil also has some antibacterial properties.

- Get comfortable. You are going to be spending about two hours a day sitting and pumping. Find a comfortable place to do it. Ensure you are warm enough or cool enough. Bring your phone close by or turn it off so you are not interrupted. Get yourself a glass of water or juice that is within reach. Put your feet up and relax. If you fall asleep, you won't be the only woman who has done so while pumping.

- Leave your pump set up in the location you pump. Dismantling your pump, or putting it out of the way, will just add to the time it takes to pump. Pumping is going to be part of your life, so it might as well be out for all to see. My pump never left my living room for the entire year I pumped; it didn't matter who was visiting! If you want, throw a towel over the pump so you don't notice it as much.

- Relax! Sometimes much easier said than done, however, it is important that you relax when you are pumping. If you are stressed or tense, it can interfere with your ability to let-down your milk. Think of the time you are pumping as a mental health break. Allow this time to be time for you. Read a book. Enjoy a tea. Call a friend. Do not sit and worry about the housework or whether your baby is going to wake up from his nap before you are done.

- Find something to occupy your mind: read, surf the Internet, watch television, talk on the phone. Do not bottle watch. The old adage, "A watched pot never boils", is especially true when pumping. You will begin to worry that you are not getting much milk and this will in turn inhibit your let-down, which will make you worry more! Just trust that it will happen as it should and enjoy your time doing something else.

- Massage your breasts prior to pumping. The stimulation can assist you in achieving a let-down. Or you can try massaging your breasts while you are pumping.

- Try using breast compressions when you are pumping. Hold your breast with your thumb on one side and fingers on the other and gently compress the breast. This will assist in getting out more milk and can help in clearing blocked ducts as well as preventing them.

- Take a warm shower or use warm compresses prior to pumping. The warmth can stimulate your breasts and help to achieve an easier let-down.

- Do not pump at too high a suction level. In general, you want to pump at the lowest suction level that removes milk for you. You will need to experiment to determine where this is. Each pump will be different as well, so if you change pumps, do not rely on the control knob to indicate the amount of suction. Too high a suction level will damage your nipples very quickly and make it painful to pump.

- Ensure that you have flanges that fit your nipples. Flange diameters range from 21 mm to 30.5 mm. If you are experiencing sore nipples or areolas, consider the size of your flange. You may need a smaller or larger flange. If you are unsure, contact a lactation consultant or your local health unit and ask for a consultation.

- Go hands free if you want. You can purchase pumping bras designed to hold the flanges in the bra, allowing you to use your hands for other things. Or you can make one yourself by taking a snug fitting bra and cutting slits in it to allow you to slip the flanges inside. This can be especially useful if you want to read, surf the Internet, or play with your baby while you are pumping. Some women become extremely adept at balancing collection bottles on their knees, allowing them to use their hands, but a pumping bra makes this unnecessary.

- Do not wear underwire bras or tight, constrictive bras. These can cause blocked ducts and impact your supply.

Over time, you will discover the method of pumping that works best for you. Until you establish your own method, here's a good strategy to begin pumping:

When starting your pumping session, start with a low suction level and high number of cycles (this is assuming the pump you are using will allow you to adjust both; some will not). If you have been breastfeeding, try to mimic your baby's sucking pattern. Once you start letting-down, decrease the cycle speed and increase the suction. This mimics the way a baby nurses: quick sucks to initiate the milk flow and then longer and stronger draws.

There are a couple breast pumps currently available that have this type of pumping program automatically built in. While this may be a good feature for many women, look for a pump that will allow you to vary the cycles and suction yourself and individualize your pumping session.

The Milk Ejection Reflex

It is important for you to release your milk when pumping and the milk ejection reflex (MER) is what causes this to happen. The MER, also called let-down, happens when a wave of oxytocin causes the cells around your alveoli to contract initiating the ejection of milk from your breasts. Women will experience the MER differently: some will never notice it at all, some will experience some slight tingling and a sensation of their breasts filling up, and some will experience what they would describe as mild pain or discomfort. It is also possible for the sensation to decrease as time goes on. As with most things, it is very individual and there is a wide range of normal.

Often the sight of your baby or the sound of his cry will initiate the MER when you are breastfeeding, however, when pumping this may not be the case. Your body will become conditioned to different things and you need your body to become conditioned to initiating the MER when you are pumping. Being relaxed, taking a warm shower before pumping, looking at a picture of your baby (or your baby for that matter), massaging your breasts before you pump and while you are pumping, and doing something while you pump other than watching your collection bottles and wishing they would fill faster will all assist in experiencing easier let-downs.

Since the MER is in some ways a conditioned response, try to maintain a similar routine when you are pumping: sit in the same location, do the same thing while pumping, listen to the same music. You will also want to limit, as much as possible, things which can impact the MER including stress, fatigue, embarrassment, cold, pain, smoking, caffeine, alcohol, and some medications.

Initiating Your Milk Supply by Pumping

When initiating your supply by pumping, frequency is key. You should aim to pump approximately every two hours around the clock if possible, with one longer stretch in the night. It is important that you pump at least once between 1 a.m. and 5 a.m. since during this time your prolactin levels are at their highest. Your goal should be to pump at least eight times within a twenty-four hour period. Until your milk "comes in", you will not be removing milk from your breasts, only colostrum. It is not necessary to pump for excessively long periods during this time. Ten to fifteen minute sessions should suffice. Remember that frequent pumping at this point is what is most important. Try not to go longer than three hours between pumps during the day when first starting to pump.

Do not attempt to cut back on this stage of pumping. What you do now will lay the groundwork for your supply down the road.

During the first few days post-partum, you will not have any mature milk to feed your baby. It can take up to seven days or more for your milk to "come in". However, this does not mean that you are not pumping anything of value for your baby. You will be pumping colostrum- a thick, yellow liquid that is rich in antibodies and immune boosting elements. Feed every drop of this to your baby. The best way to collect it is with a syringe which can then be used to feed it to your child. You can, during this period, supplement with formula if you wish. However, remember that breastfed babies would not be receiving anything but colostrum from their mothers, and there is no need to supplement breastfed babies at this stage in their lives unless there are medical complications that require supplementation. Your baby will have the desire to suckle though, so if you are not breastfeeding you should consider the use of a pacifier.

Once your milk supply starts to increase, continue to pump every two to three hours with at least one session between 1 a.m. and 5 a.m.. Information from numerous women who exclusively pump indicates that women pump on average about 120 minutes within a twenty-four hour period. This guideline of 120 minutes will continue to be valid for as long as you pump; every time you drop a pump, you will add time to your sessions to ensure you are pumping for approximately 120 minutes every day.

As you continue to pump, gauge your schedule by your supply. You will want to establish, if possible, a daily volume that exceeds the maximum daily intake of your baby at his highest intake level. You may decide you want to have a very large supply, or you may need a larger supply if you are pumping for multiples. However, keep in mind that the larger your supply, the lower the fat content in your milk. This is especially important to consider if you are pumping for a premature infant or an infant for whom weight gain is an issue. Unless you are only planning on pumping for a short amount of time and want to freeze as much milk as possible, you may want to prevent your supply from growing too large (in excess of 1500 milliliters/day or 50 ounces/day).

Considering that most babies' maximum daily milk intake will be around 960 milliliters a day (thirty-two ounces), a volume in excess of this maximum will rarely be required. Establishing a supply to around 1200-1500 milliliters (forty or fifty ounces) will allow for ample milk to freeze and should cover any drop in supply that may occur when dropping pumping sessions. But it will ensure you do not have too many issues with excessive milk storage, low fat content, or engorgement. But once again, all this is very individual. Some women will maintain a very consistent volume regardless of their pumping routine, while others notice significant decreases as they change their schedule. In my opinion, it is best to be prepared for decreases rather than worrying about not having enough expressed milk to feed your baby.

Some women may not reach this volume, in which case you will want to continue with the initial schedule until you reach about two or three months post-partum. If you do decide to drop a session earlier than this, you run the risk of affecting your supply down the road. While this is not an absolute, you unfortunately will not know until it is too late. It is best to take advantage of your high prolactin levels while you have them.

If your supply does reach a suitable volume, or you reach approximately the two to three month mark, you should be at a point where you can safely start to drop pumping sessions (unless you have an extremely low supply in which case it is best to continue to pump often). Drop them slowly! No more than one a month is a good guideline. Of course, the rate at which you drop pumps will also be determined by when you want to wean. In general, the longer you want to pump, the slower you should drop pumping sessions.

When deciding on which pumping session to drop, consider that the night pump is still the period of highest prolactin levels in your body. Maintaining this pumping session can be of benefit to your volumes. That being said, most women decide to drop this pumping session once their babies start to sleep through the night. However, it is best to wait until two or three months post-partum to drop the night pump. I personally continued to pump during the night for nine months although my son started to sleep through the night around six months. I found this allowed me to have more time through the day between pumps and gave me more time to spend with my son. This schedule worked for me but wasn't necessary. Decide what you will do based on your individual needs and situation.

Switching to Exclusively Pumping after Breastfeeding

If you have established your supply breastfeeding, the switch to exclusively pumping will require a similar schedule to the one outlined above regardless of how long you were breastfeeding. You will start pumping using 120 minutes per day of pumping as a guideline. There are a few reasons for this:

- Your body will respond to a pump differently than it responded to your baby. You will need to "retrain" your body. You may find that your milk ejection reflex is not as reliable as with your baby, and therefore, it will take longer to remove your breast milk with a pump.

- Your baby may be better at emptying your breasts than a pump. Therefore, while your baby may maintain your supply only feeding five times a day, you may not find this the case with a pump, and you will need to pump more frequently than if you were breastfeeding.

- Since when you are exclusively pumping you will find it more difficult to increase your supply later on, and since your young infant is not yet close to her maximum daily intake, you will want to increase your supply now in order to allow yourself the ability to drop pumps later.

When making the switch from breastfeeding to exclusively pumping, pump every two to three hours during the day and at least once between 1 a.m. and 5 a.m.. Aim for at least six to eight sessions within a twenty-four hour period. The lower your supply and the younger your baby, the more often you will want to pump. Ensure you are pumping approximately 120 minutes a day.

My recommendation is to continue to pump at this schedule until your supply exceeds the maximum daily intake that your baby will require (approximately 960 milliliters or thirty-two ounces). If you do produce a high volume, you may attempt to drop a pumping session, but if you are not pumping a high volume, maintain this schedule as long as you can or until you reach at least two to three months post-partum.

Remember, for the first month or two post-partum you have high levels of prolactin assisting you with milk production. Use this to your advantage and establish as strong a supply as you can within this time period.

By two to three months post-partum, lactation switches to the autocrine process- milk removed means more milk produced. You can not rely on your pump to remove milk as well as your baby. This is why it is harder to increase your supply after three months- but not impossible.

Individual Considerations

Women will empty their breasts at different rates. Some women have a stronger MER than others. Keep in mind that everyone is different and some women will need to pump longer and some women will find they can maintain a supply pumping less. Also, different pumps will affect the length of time needed to empty the breast; some will be more effective than others. Take the time recommendations offered here as a guideline, and do alter them for your individual situation if need be.

Also, it is important to understand that the MER is not continuous. Oxytocin, which initiates the MER, is not continuously present. It is released in waves. Therefore, just because your milk flow stops does not mean that you have emptied your breasts sufficiently. If you continue to breastfeed or pump, you will in most cases experience another let-down. In fact, the common belief that you can empty your breasts is a misconception. Milk is continually produced, making it impossible to completely empty your breasts. Therefore, the often heard advice to pump until your milk stops flowing is not necessarily good advice to maintain a strong supply. Watching the clock, maintaining accurate records, and adding time to your pumping sessions as you drop pumps to constantly achieve at least 120 minutes of pumping each day is probably a far better strategy.

Maintaining Your Supply

The key to maintaining your supply for the long-term is to create an environment that will allow for optimal milk production and remove the milk from your breasts. It is that simple. What is not simple, however, is controlling all the variables that can affect your supply, having the stamina to continue a rigorous pumping schedule, and continuing to spend time with your pump instead of your baby. Regardless, the key to maintaining a strong supply is to ensure the milk in your breasts is removed regularly ensuring the feedback loop signals for more milk to be produced. An excellent breast pump is an absolute necessity, but beyond the pump, there are a number of things you can do to both build a strong supply and maintain it. If your supply declines after a few weeks or months, it is sometimes possible to increase it, but not always.

It is best not lose your supply in the first place! Be sure to:

- Maintain a good pumping schedule. After taking care of your baby, pumping sessions must take priority in your day. There is no quick fix for a haphazard schedule. Remember you want to aim for around 120 minutes a day. While you do not need to pump at exactly the same time every day, you should aim for the same number of sessions every day and try not to go any longer than six hours between pumping sessions.

- Do not drop pumping sessions too early. It is very tempting to drop sessions as quickly as possible, but you don't know how this will affect you long-term. Remember that early on, it is frequency and stimulation that will establish your supply and impact your ability to pump long-term. Do not be hasty. The extra effort early on will pay off in the long run.

- Reduce the stress in your life when possible. Stress can quickly reduce your milk supply and is one of the most common supply reducers. Make time for yourself, if possible, to engage in stress reducing activities. Relax your expectations and accept help when it's offered.

Share your stress with your friends and partner; let them share the load.

- Eat well. Caloric and carbohydrate intake drastically affect the fat content of your milk. Your vitamin and mineral intake also directly affect the milk you produce. Be sure you are eating a healthy variety and eating enough. While you do not need to eat a great deal more when lactating than you normally would, you do need to ensure a consistent level of nourishment. Now is not the time to diet.

- Drink enough water. The key here is to not become dehydrated. You do not need to drink excessive amounts of water. In fact, some information suggests too much water can have a negative impact on your supply. Drink the recommended 8-10 glasses of water each day and try to avoid coffees and sodas which can dehydrate you.

- Avoid the use of hormonal birth control containing estrogen. The use of a progestin-only oral contraceptive is preferred if you wish to take birth control pills, however, wait until your supply is well established before starting them. Always monitor your supply closely if you do start any new medications in case it has a negative impact on your supply.

- Avoid the use of antihistamines. While there is no conclusive verification showing that antihistamines have a negative impact on milk supply, there has been anecdotal evidence suggesting that this can result. Antihistamines do pass into breast milk, however, so it is probably best to avoid them for this reason alone.

- Carefully research any medication or herbal supplement before taking to find out both its effects on lactation and whether it is passed on to the baby through your milk. Motherisk, operated from The Hospital for Sick Children in Toronto, is an excellent resource. They offer extensive information on pregnancy and drug use; breastfeeding and drug use; prescription and over the counter medications; as well as tobacco, alcohol, and illegal drugs. www.motherisk.org

- Use an excellent quality double electric hospital-grade breast pump. There is no better method to establishing and maintaining a strong supply when pumping than using the best possible breast pump. If you are not finding success, consider trying a different pump for a trial period to see if it makes a difference.

Supplementing With Formula

Some women will never require any type of intervention or alternative strategies for increasing or maintaining their milk supply. They pump, and they produce ample amounts of milk for their baby's daily needs with enough left over to build up a significant freezer stash. However, some women will not find a sufficient supply so easy to come by. For these women, their milk volume will constantly be a source of concern, barely maintaining enough to feed their baby or perhaps not producing enough at all.

While most women who exclusively pump want to provide 100% breast milk for their child, this is not always going to happen. In some cases, supplementation with commercially prepared formula will be necessary. But remember that any amount of breast milk is beneficial, and although your baby might not be receiving all his nourishment from your milk, he is receiving all the benefits of your breast milk.

When supplementing with formula, it is best to feed bottles of breast milk and bottles of formula separately. There are a number of reasons for this:

- The anti-infective properties of breast milk may be reduced by combining it with formula (Quan R. et al., Clinical Pediatrics, 1994).

- The components of the formula can interfere with the absorption of the iron in your breast milk.

- Once you mix breast milk and formula, you must then treat it as you would formula which means if it is not finished within an hour, it must be discarded. For women who are struggling to produce every drop, it can be heartbreaking to throw out any amount of breast milk. In this case, feed breast milk and formula separately.

Having said that, many women do mix formula and breast milk. There is no danger in doing it. It is perfectly safe and sometimes may be necessary or preferred. Mixing formula and breast milk is also a helpful method of switching a baby onto formula when weaning.

There is absolutely no reason to be discouraged about supplementing with formula. Many mothers supplement at one time or another- both pumping mothers and breastfeeding mothers. Keep working on increasing your supply, but recognize that your baby is still benefiting from your dedication to pump.

Ways to Increase Your Supply

If you are not able to initiate a sufficient supply, or your supply has decreased, consider the following possible reasons for a low supply or decreased supply and strategies and techniques for boosting your supply:

- Do you possibly have a blocked duct or mastitis? Both can dramatically reduce your supply. See the chapter entitled "Overcoming Difficulties" for symptoms and treatments.

- Are you getting enough sleep? Although sleep and babies do not always go together, it is important that you are as rested as possible. Can someone else take care of the baby for awhile so you can rest? Could you hire a babysitter so you can get some shut-eye?

- Is your pump working as it should? Take your pump apart and check for any tears in the membranes, holes in the tubing, or blockages. Listen to the pump's motor: does it sound like it is working well? Put the flange up to your cheek and turn the pump on. Does it create suction? If you are concerned it may be your pump reducing your supply, call the pump manufacturer. See

"Resources" for the web sites of major pump manufacturers.

- Have you recently started taking any type of medication, either prescription or non-prescription? Check to see if this medication could possibly reduce your milk supply. While you may have checked to see if it was safe for your baby, you might have overlooked the effects on lactation.

- Ensure you are receiving adequate nutrition. While lactation will happen regardless of what you eat, poor diet can impact you in numerous other ways. It can cause you to get run-down leading to illness, it can impact your ability to handle stress, and it can affect your overall sense of well-being. Your milk supply *may* decrease if you are not taking in enough calories; although, the fat content of your milk *will* be adversely affected. If your milk has a low fat content, your baby will need more milk to meet her caloric needs. If your supply is also reduced, this is going to create a problem. Sufficient calories and carbohydrates are a definite must.

- Drink 8-10 glasses of water a day. As already mentioned, you do not need extra water, just ensure you are not getting dehydrated.

- Try eating oatmeal daily. Many women give anecdotal support to the value of oatmeal to increase their milk supply. Oatmeal in any form will work- even oatmeal cookies! Consider starting your day with a bowl of hot oatmeal. Some mothers also drink de-alcoholized beer reporting similar effects.

- Herbal supplements such as fenugreek and Mother's Milk Tea help some women increase their supply. These should not be taken together, however, since Mother's Milk Tea contains fenugreek. In addition to fenugreek, Mother's Milk Tea also contains sweet fennel seed, anise seed, coriander seed, spearmint leaf, lemongrass leaf, lemon verbena leaf, althea root, and blessed thistle herb. Fenugreek smells like maple syrup, and if you take enough of it, you too will smell like maple syrup.

Fenugreek has also been associated with gassiness and stomach irritability in both mother and baby, so be watchful for those symptoms.

- Reducing the stress in your life as much as possible will assist your efforts to increase and maintain your supply. Many women find that when they are highly stressed, they have a marked decrease in their daily milk volume. Avoid it when you can, deal with it in healthy ways when you can't. Try exercising, find a support group either in your community or online, journal daily to release emotions, pray, and lean on those around you who care about you.

- Have you started taking hormonal birth control or have you recently started your period? Hormones can play havoc with your milk supply. While your supply will usually improve after your period ends, it might not always pick back up to its former volume. If you find your period returns while still pumping and your supply decreases just prior to and during your period, try taking calcium and magnesium supplements. The suggested dosage on Kellymom.com is between 500 mg calcium and 250 mg magnesium to 1500 mg calcium and 750 mg magnesium. It is best to start taking the supplements about one week prior to the beginning of your period and taking it throughout.

- Domperidone and metoclopramide are prescription drugs which many have found helpful to increase milk supply. Both drugs are best used for mothers of premature babies who are having difficulty establishing a supply; however, they can be used by mothers who are not pumping sufficient volumes for their babies. These drugs should only be considered when all other options have been exhausted. Both metoclopramide and domperidone increase the levels of prolactin in the lactating mother. They will not, however, make up for poor pumping habits or allow you to pump less often.

  Many mothers report depression as a side-effect of metoclopramide (with the brand names of Reglan or Maxeran). Other possible side-effects include dizziness, nausea, sweating, and gastric cramping. If taking metoclopramide, you should start to see an increase in your supply within two or three days.

Domperidone can also be used to increase milk supply. Depression is not a side-effect associated with domperidone. It does bring with it the possibility of dry mouth, abdominal cramping, and headaches which often go away when the dosage is reduced.

It is extremely important to note that domperidone is not approved in any country for use by breastfeeding mothers in order to increase milk production. The Food and Drug Administration in the United States of America issued a release in June of 2004 warning against women using domperidone to increase their milk supply (see "Resources" for the web site address of the press release). They highlight that the distribution or importation of the drug is illegal in the U.S.A. It can, however, be obtained in the U.S.A. with a doctor's prescription filled through a compounding pharmacy.

If you are considering the use of either domperidone or metoclopramide, you need to seek the advice of a doctor who is knowledgeable about breastfeeding and the use of these drugs to increase breast milk supply.

The most important element to building and maintaining a strong milk supply is to establish and maintain excellent pumping habits!

Power Pumping and Cluster Pumping

If you need to increase your supply, there are a couple of pumping techniques you can try: power pumping or cluster pumping. Power pumping requires frequent pumping throughout the day. You should pump every two hours around the clock for at least two days. Power pumping is essentially trying to mimic a growth spurt by removing as much milk as possible and signaling your body to make more to meet the demand. There is no way to increase your supply other than removing more milk from your breasts.

Some women who power pump will spend a weekend focused on the process. They will enlist the help of family or friends to care for the baby so that they can focus on pumping frequently. Having multiple sets of flanges and lots of collection bottles so you do not need to wash and sterilize after each pumping session can also assist in making it through the rigorous power pumping schedule.

Cluster pumping is a variation on power pumping. In this case you want to be pumping frequently, as with power pumping. However, you will pump for shorter periods. For example, you will pump every half hour for ten minutes. Do this for several hours. The benefit to cluster pumping is that you can do it for only a portion of the day and then repeat it every few days. You will be very much tied down to your pump while cluster pumping, but it will not require the multiple day commitment of power pumping.

Dropping Pumping Sessions

One of the first questions new mothers will ask when they start to exclusively pump is "when can I drop a pumping session". It is best not to rush. Remember that it is the first few weeks post-partum that are crucial to establishing a strong milk supply. Dropping pumps too quickly can limit the number of prolactin receptors laid down in the breasts. And by dropping pumps too quickly in the first few months, you are not taking advantage of the naturally high prolactin levels in your body. For these reasons, it is best to wait until around three months post-partum to drop pumping sessions or until you have established a strong supply as previously discussed.

Yet, some women do choose to drop pumping sessions earlier than three months. It is highly individual as to when it is advisable or perhaps simply necessary for a person's sanity to drop a pump. Keep in mind your long-term goals and the current daily volume that you are pumping. There is no guarantee as to what dropping a pump will do to your supply. You will have to judge it based on your knowledge of lactation, your supply, and your ability to continue pumping.

The most common reason a woman gives for dropping a pumping session is the need to regain time in her life: to take back some of what pumping has taken away. This time might be used to sleep, to spend with family, to care for the baby, or a number of other things, but time is what pumping can take away from you and is what most women want to regain. I firmly believe that women know when they need to drop a pump. You will just get to a point where it has to be done to maintain a balance. Trust your instincts and be comfortable in your decision before you drop the pumping session. Understand that it may negatively affect your supply, and if it does, there is a possibility that you will not be able to regain lost volume.

While some women will see an increase in supply when they drop a pumping session, others will see a decrease. This has a lot to do with a woman's storage capacity. If a woman has a large capacity, she often sees an increase in supply simply because she has a longer period of time to produce milk and the capacity to store it- remember the breast is continually producing milk. However, those women with a smaller storage capacity will have to pump more often to achieve the same volumes. Once you understand whether you have a large or small storage capacity, you will better be able to gauge how quickly you can drop pumps and be able to know how few pumping sessions you can do per day without starting to lose your supply.

When dropping a pumping session you have three options:

1. You can drop an actual session and continue pumping the remaining sessions at their usual times. For example if you usually pump at 7a.m., 10 a.m., 1 p.m., 4p.m., 7p.m., 10p.m., and 2 a.m., you may want to drop the 10 a.m. pumping session. Simply dropping the session will allow you a longer stretch of time in the day without having to pump. You may find however, that you get quite engorged having such a long period between pumps. You may want to pump a little earlier and reduce the length of time between pumps slightly to accommodate your discomfort. Do not allow yourself to get extremely engorged to the point of pain. This will only lead to blocked ducts or mastitis. If you are prone to blocks or mastitis, you may be best dropping pumps by the next method.

2. The second way to drop a pumping session is to simply lengthen the length of time between all your pumping sessions. For example, if you had been pumping every three hours, extend this to every four hours. You may need to pump once or twice after only three hours to fit in all your sessions. An example of this new schedule might be 7 a.m., 11 a.m., 3 p.m., 6 p.m., 10 p.m., and 2 p.m..

3. The third option is to not worry about how long you wait between pumping sessions but instead to pump where and when you can. It is the number of pumping sessions per day as well as the total pumping time throughout the day that is most important. Aim for approximately 120 minutes per day of pumping. Most women find that their volume remains consistent regardless of how long they may go between pumping sessions. If you are trying to pump five times a day, it will make little difference if you pump at 6 a.m., 11 a.m., 4 p.m., 10 p.m., and 3 a.m., or pump at 6 a.m., 9 a.m., 1 p.m., 3 p.m., 9 p.m., and 2 a.m.. Both schedules should provide you will the same volumes.

The following are important guidelines when dropping pumping sessions:

- It is best not go any more than six hours between pumping sessions. Remember that the longer milk stays in the breast, the slower production becomes. This is obviously going to be disregarded when you drop down to three pumping sessions a day.

- Do not drop the night pump before you reach approximately three months post-partum. You should be pumping at least once between 1 a.m. and 5 a.m.. Your prolactin levels are at their highest at night. Take advantage of them. After approximately three months, your prolactin levels start to decline, and this night pump is not as important although continuing to pump at night can still be beneficial to a low supply.

- Go slowly when dropping pumping sessions. Consider your long-term goals (the longer your goal, the more slowly you will want to drop sessions). Allow yourself enough time to recognize any negative trends in your supply before you think about dropping another session. A good general guideline is to not drop any more than one session per month (unless of course you want to wean).

Beyond Establishing Your Supply

Once you are on your way to establishing your supply and have your initial schedule down, you may start to question your choice to exclusively pump: was this the right decision? Can I really keep this up? You may be feeling overwhelmed, and you are most definitely exhausted. Now is a good time to step back, look at the big picture, and set some goals.

How long do you plan to pump?

Those women who are able to make it past the first few difficult months are often surprised that they end up exclusively pumping longer than they had even planned to breastfeed. Once able to drop pumping sessions to a more manageable level, everything tends to become routine and the prospect of continuing more probable.

Set small, achievable goals and work towards those. Keep your sights on the goal date, and manage day-by-day and even pump-by-pump if necessary. Soon you will meet your goal and at that time you can reassess:

- Do you want to continue pumping?
- How is your supply?
- Do you feel you will be able to continue both physically and mentally?
- Do you have your family's support?

The answers to these questions will play into your decision to either continue or wean. If you decide to continue, set a new goal and go for it! If you decide to wean, review how to wean in the chapter "Weaning" and take it slowly. Depending on how much breast milk you are currently pumping, you should allow yourself between two and four weeks to wean comfortably.

If your supply is not meeting your baby's needs and you are thinking about weaning, you may want to consider supplementing with formula to make up the short-fall as an alternative. Any amount of breast milk is beneficial to your child, and breast milk is still far superior to formula. While your baby may not receive 100% breast milk, she does receive 100% of the benefits of your milk. You will need to decide what is best for your baby, but realize that pumping does not have to be an all or nothing proposition if your supply is on the lower end of the scale.

Often once women meet their long-term goal, they pump on a day-to-day basis, meaning that they take every day pumping as a bonus to their baby. My long-term goal was eight months, when my son would be six months adjusted in age. After reaching this point, I felt very little stress about pumping, knowing that mentally I would be comfortable weaning when I felt ready.

Creating a Balance

For many women, it is easy to become consumed with pumping. Everything, it seems, becomes focused on providing breast milk for your baby. Often this is because mothers feel guilty about not being able to breastfeed and are determined to make pumping work. This focus, however, can create an imbalance in your life and cause problems within your marriage, with your health, or your overall well-being. It is very important to attempt to look at the larger picture (which admittedly can be difficult) and take active steps to create balance in your life and home:

- Speak openly with your spouse. Explain the importance of feeding breast milk to your baby- both the medical benefits to you and your baby and the emotional benefits to you. Enlist his support and understanding. Accept his help. Listen to his concerns. Often a husband's suggestions to wean early are due to concern for you and your own health and well-being. Suggest concrete ways that he can support you such as taking the baby for an afternoon while you catch up on rest or making dinners once in a while or even massaging your feet while you pump.

- Let go of assumptions and expectations. Accept things as they are. Take things as they come. Be willing to bend. Things rarely work out as we expect them. You may have expected to breastfeed. You may have expected to have everything in your household under control. Things change. Don't worry about how you thought things were going to be. Focus instead on what you do have and the situation you are now in.

- Find someone to share your feelings and concerns with. Talk it out! Pumping can sometimes be very isolating since it often contains you in your home, especially early on. Get support- a friend, an online discussion board (see "Resources" for a list of online discussion boards), a doctor, a lactation consultant, your mother- anyone who you trust and who is interested in listening, understanding, and supporting.

- Think through worst-case scenarios. What is the worst thing that would happen if you quit pumping? Or lost your supply? Or had to start supplementing with formula? This will either spur you on or give yourself permission to relax a little and recognize that the alternative isn't so bad.

- If you are running on empty, consider dropping a pumping session. The reason most women give for dropping a session is the need to get back some time to do things through the day; to sleep more; or to have more time with the baby, other children or their spouse.

Don't allow pumping to affect your health, your relationship with your baby, or your relationship with your spouse. Keep things in balance.

How much milk do you really need to pump?

The volume of milk a woman is able to pump on a daily basis will vary from individual to individual. However, the stronger your supply early on, the more options you will have later in terms of dropping pumping sessions and the freedom to consider weaning before your goal date while continuing to feed frozen breast milk. When it comes right down to it, what truly matters is that you are able to feed your baby expressed breast milk, regardless of whether you may need to supplement with formula or not.

As discussed in the previous chapter, the storage capacity of a woman's breasts has an impact when exclusively pumping. Women with a smaller storage capacity may find they need to pump more often than a woman with a larger storage capacity. It is for this reason that you must approach exclusively pumping from an individual perspective. Do not attempt to follow a prescriptive approach. Take all information as guidelines that may need to be altered for each individual. However, do understand the science of lactation - this can not be altered!

Women with large storage capacities may be able to pump as little as two or three times a day and still completely meet the needs of their child- or exceed them. But, women with smaller storage capacities may find if they attempt to drop to only two or three pumps a day, they will start to lose supply and initiate a weaning process.

Keep track of your daily volumes. Record this information daily and review it often to note trends. Some women will create and maintain a spreadsheet of this information. This information is especially important when you drop pumping sessions. It will highlight very quickly if you are starting on a downward trend in terms of your supply. For those women with larger capacities, your records may indicate that your supply increases when dropping sessions.

While it is important to keep track of your daily volumes, try not to get too caught up in the numbers. Remember you are doing all of this for your baby, and becoming obsessed with these numbers will only add more stress to your life. Your volumes will fluctuate on a daily basis. When looking at your volumes, look for trends over the course of a few days.

Numerous things can cause fluctuations in your supply such as dehydration, lack of sleep, or too much stress. Very rarely will these cause any long-term concerns provided you change the root cause of the fluctuation. Breastfeeding mothers have fluctuations as well, but as long as their babies are satisfied, they rarely notice.

If you do find a downward trend in your volume over a period of a few days, start some investigative work to try and determine the cause. See the chapter "Fundamentals of Exclusively Pumping" for a list of possible causes of supply decrease and methods to increase supply.

The length of time you intend to pump also impacts the kind of volume you will want to initiate. In my opinion, the longer you plan on pumping, the larger the supply you initially want. The reason for this is that when you drop pumping sessions- and you will want to drop them- it is safest to assume you will lose some of your daily volume. Some women will see an increase with the first few sessions they drop due primarily to a large breast storage capacity, but you won't know if this will be your experience until you actually drop sessions.

While a breastfeeding mother can rely on her baby to increase her supply by feeding more frequently and for longer periods when the baby requires more milk, mothers who are exclusively pumping would have to do this by pumping more often and for longer periods. Very few women will want to do this after a few months when the baby's appetite increases and after having dropped a pumping session or two. Therefore, starting with a stronger supply will cushion any drop in volume you may experience when dropping pumps. A larger supply early on will also allow you to freeze excess milk to cushion any drops in volume later on, and it may allow you to continue feeding breast milk even after you wean.

However, if you have a shorter goal, you may not ever require high volumes of breast milk and 750-900 milliliters (twenty-five to thirty ounces) a day may be enough for your baby for the first three months or more (it would have satisfied my son for his entire first year). Remember though, it will be much more difficult to increase your supply later on, and since no one ever knows what the future holds, it is best, in my opinion, to build as strong a supply as possible in the beginning. This will allow you more flexibility while pumping and give you the option of continuing past your original goal date or feeding frozen milk past your weaning date.

Look At the Big Picture

When discussing volumes, it is important to step back and get a look at the big picture. Exclusively pumping is hard work. It can be exhausting. And while it is done to provide the very best for your baby, it is important not to forget about another important element a baby requires- a loving mother who is able to respond to her baby's needs.

Work to maintain a balance between establishing and maintaining your supply and maintaining a life that allows you to establish a strong, loving bond with your baby. If you feel like you can't continue as you are, try dropping a pumping session and see what happens. Remember, though, that it is advisable not to drop a session until your supply is well established. Once you have a good grasp of the fundamentals of pumping and the science of lactation, you will be able to make an educated decision and understand the possible ramifications of your choices.

As well, do not make a rash decision to drop a pump. Ensure you are not making the decision out of frustration, anger, or fatigue. Often it is best to wait a few days after deciding to drop a session before you actually cut it out of your schedule. Set yourself a goal date when you plan on dropping the pump. Once you get to that date, if you still feel it is time to do it and you need to do it, then go ahead and drop it. Do it to maintain a balance in your health, your relationships, your life.

Every woman who exclusively pumps has days where she does not think she can continue. You will not be the first and you will not be the last. Look at the larger picture. Think about why you are doing what you are doing. Weigh the pros and cons. Understand what your options are and how they might affect your long-term goal. Be honest with yourself about your emotions and strive to maintain a balance. Some days you might have to take one pump at a time; throw that long-term goal out the window for the day. Chances are tomorrow things will look better. But if they don't, it's okay to do what you need to do. Trust yourself and know that you have a lot more determination and strength now that you are a mother. If you want to do it, you will find a way.

You're Feeding Your Baby, Not the Freezer

Often, women who are exclusively pumping become focused on freezing as much milk as possible. Seeing frozen breast milk in the freezer is in many ways tangible proof of your hard work and provides a safety net in case of a supply disaster. A complete change in mindset occurred for me after approximately five months of pumping when someone on the Exclusively Pumping discussion board at iVillage reminded me that I was pumping to feed my baby, not my freezer.

Up to this point, I was producing far more than my son required. Having been nine weeks premature, I had a very large head start on him in terms of my supply and his intake. Within two months, my small apartment-sized freezer was overflowing. I was constantly stressing about where to put the large amount of breast milk I was pumping every day. I was planning to begin rotating my freezer stash: start feeding frozen breast milk and freezing my fresh milk. But I knew that fresh milk was the best for my baby. After all, why was I going through all the trials of pumping if not to feed my son the best possible?

It was a response to my post on the message board asking for advice about my growing freezer stash, limited freezer space, and the desire to feed my son the best possible, when I was reminded that I was doing all this to feed my baby, not my freezer. This comment helped me to regain a balance, gain perspective on my situation, and perhaps made it possible for me to pump for another seven months. From that moment on, I fed my son exclusively fresh milk and culled my freezer stash when necessary to allow me to freeze more fresh milk. I was comfortable knowing that my son was getting the best expressed breast milk possible for as long as I chose to pump and knew that I would still have some frozen milk to feed after I weaned.

Low Volume Producers

If you are a low volume producer, then the discussion of freezing milk and dealing with the large volumes produced will undoubtedly leave you feeling a little disappointed, upset, or frustrated. Do not despair. As has been said previously, any amount of breast milk is beneficial and even though your baby may not be receiving 100% breast milk, he is receiving 100% of the benefit from your breast milk. Many women who do not pump enough for their baby choose to supplement with formula instead of weaning. This is a decision that will have to be made by you.

Think about your pumping habits and the pump you are using. Can you find a cause for your low volume? Is it possible that you can increase your supply by improving your pumping habits or using a better pump? But start now- don't let poor pumping habits continue any longer.

If you have tried everything and still are not producing the volume you would like, then you will perhaps just have to accept it. Feel proud of yourself for having the courage and determination to continue pumping! You are showing true dedication to your baby to provide her with breast milk, and the amount you pump truly has no bearing on the gift you are giving your baby.

Breast Pumps, Kits, and Accessories

One of the most important factors to successful pumping is the pump you choose to use. In order to build and maintain a strong supply, you must remove the breast milk from your breasts- this is an absolute. A baby is by far the most efficient pump you can find, but when you must choose a mechanical breast pump, all pumps are not created equal.

A significant difference has been shown in the ability of various breast pumps to produce a strong prolactin response in lactating mothers. The best type of breast pump was found to be an electric pulsatile breast pump (Zinamen, M. et al., Pediatrics, 1992). As well, a distinct increase in the production of breast milk has been seen when double pumping was utilized by the pumping mother compared to single pumping (Jones, E., Archives of Disease in Childhood Neonatal Edition, 2001).

After investigating the research that has been conducted on breast pumps, an understanding of what to look for when buying or renting a breast pump can be formulated. An electric pump that allows you to adjust both the suction level as well as the number of cycles it pumps is preferred and will allow you to individualize the pump to meet your own needs. It is vitally important that you use a pump that will allow you to pump both breasts at the same time; not only will this save you time, but it can increase your milk volume. Another important consideration is the purpose for which the pump was originally created. There are many good breast pumps on the market; however, many of these were not intended for the extended and frequent use of a woman exclusively pumping. While they might do a satisfactory job for a while, it is possible that the motor may be over-taxed and result in decreased performance which in turn will result in decreased supply for you, or they simply may not provide enough stimulation to initiate and maintain a strong supply.

It is also important that a breast pump supplies the right amount of suction and the right number of suck and release cycles per minute. A breastfeeding baby creates between 40 and 60 suck and release cycles per minute and a baby's maximum suction is around 200 to 220 mm Hg (millimeters of Mercury which is a measure of pressure). While many breast pumps do fall within these ranges, there are a number that do not. Before settling on a pump, find out the specifications for the pump. Choose one that will provide the cycles and suction as closely resembling a baby as possible. An excellent Internet resource comparing the specifications of most breast pumps can be found at www.leron-line.com/updates/Breast_Pumps.htm.

The best advice is to use the best breast pump you can afford. Consider the cost of feeding formula for six months or a year, and in most cases you will discover that even the most expensive breast pump is a great value. And when you factor in the enormous benefits of breast milk for your baby in terms of health and development, you will recognize what a great bargain a breast pump truly is.

Almost all baby product companies have a breast pump among their product offerings. However, many of these pumps are very inefficient and may not even serve a breastfeeding mother very well. Often, these pumps are offered simply to complete a product line or to position the company as being breastfeeding friendly while the majority of their profits come from bottle feeding and formula feeding supplies. Beware of these pumps if you are exclusively pumping!

Instead, look for a company that focuses primarily on breast pumps and breastfeeding. These companies will continually strive to improve their products and conduct research that will benefit pumping moms. Companies that fit into this description are Medela, Hollister/Ameda, Avent, Whittlestone, and Bailey Medical. However, while these companies focus their efforts to support breastfeeding and breastfeeding mothers, this does not mean that all of their breast pumps will be suitable for an exclusively pumping mother.

Before making a decision on a breast pump, learn about your options. Read the rest of this chapter. Go on-line and search for more information about breast pumps. Talk to a lactation consultant for her recommendations. Go to the Internet discussion boards listed at the end of this book and find out what other pumping moms are using. Rent a pump and see if it works for you. Most importantly, choose a pump that will provide strong enough suction while being able to withstand the rigors of exclusive pumping.

Open Vs. Closed Milk Collection Systems

Breast pumps operate on either an open system or a closed system. An open system means that there is no barrier between the milk and the tubing, and therefore the motor, of the pump. In a closed system, there is a barrier in place that prevents any contact between the milk and the tubing and other internal parts of the pump.

All hospital-grade pumps work on a closed system allowing the pump to be used by multiple women without fear of cross-contamination. However, not all personal pumps work on a closed system. If purchasing your own new breast pump, the fact of whether the pump has an open or closed system really does not impact you as long as you keep your pump and kit well maintained. However, an open system breast pump is not one that should be used by multiple women. These pumps are single-user pumps and do run the risk of contaminating breast milk if used by more than one woman. It is strongly recommended that you do not purchase or borrow a previously used open system breast pump.

There are a couple companies that do offer personal breast pumps that can be safely used by multiple users. Ameda pumps use what they call a HygieniKit. This kit has a patented silicone diaphragm which prevents milk particles from entering the tubing or motor, thereby protecting subsequent users of the breast pump. Bailey Medical's Nurture III breast pump is also advertised as being safe for multiple users. For each pump, each woman must use her own collection kit.

Types of Pumps

Manual Breast Pumps

Manual pumps are just as the name suggests- powered manually. Most work with a piston that you pump in order to create suction; however, models such as the Avent Isis and the Medela Harmony use a hand trigger. Many manual pumps do allow the user to vary the suction level. The cycling is determined by your operation. Manual pumps can only be used to pump one breast at a time. They are convenient to travel with since they are small and compact. One drawback of hand pumps is the possibility of repetitive strain injuries to the hand and wrist if a manual pump is used frequently. They can also be awkward to use since both hands must be used to hold the pump and/or the breast.

While there are a few cases in which women have successfully exclusively pumped long-term with a hand pump, these success stories are not the norm. It is important to note that manual pumping is far more time consuming since you are only able to single pump, and the effort it takes to manually operate the pump will make it more difficult to continue indefinitely. In the vast majority of cases, a manual pump is not an option for exclusively pumping.

A manual pump may, however, be a useful back-up pump for emergencies or the occasional outing.

Battery Operated and Small Electric Breast Pumps

These pumps are often ones bearing the name of large baby product companies and are most commonly found in drug and department stores. Often, these are the companies that have developed a breast pump in order to offer a complete range of infant products. They most commonly will only allow single-sided pumping and many mothers report that they are uncomfortable to use. While these pumps may be acceptable for infrequent use by a breastfeeding mother, they will not initiate or maintain a milk supply when exclusively pumping.

These pumps are very inexpensive when compared to the better quality single-user pumps or hospital-grade pumps, but do not be seduced by the price- they will not meet your needs!

Single-User Electric Breast Pumps

There are a number of manufacturers that offer electric breast pumps for single-users: Medela, Hollister/Ameda, and Bailey Medical. These pumps are intended to only be used by one person and are not intended to be resold or loaned out since some do not operate on a closed system and they are not built to withstand the rigors of multiple users.

Many women have exclusively pumped successfully with this type of pump. The most commonly used pumps for exclusively pumping are the Medela Pump In Style and the Ameda Purely Yours.

The benefit to this type of pump is that they are compact, lightweight, and highly portable. Many are built into a carrying case and include cooler compartments making it very easy to pump on the go. Many of these pumps can also be used with either batteries or a car adapter that can be plugged into the cigarette lighter. Batteries, however, should not be used as a long-term option. A single pumping session can drain the batteries enough to affect the suction level of the pump for the next pumping session. Yet, if no other power source is available, the ability to use batteries is a real advantage.

These pumps can be purchased from numerous stores and from many Internet sources. The cost is notably more than the "drugstore" type of pumps, but their efficiency is far superior.

Hospital-grade Electric Pumps

The industrial hospital-grade electric pump is the best pump you can use in terms of efficiency, reliability, and durability. These pumps are often cost prohibitive to purchase outright but can be rented at a price that is usually far less than the cost of formula would be. The cost to purchase can actually still be less than formula over the course of a year and these pumps can be resold without concern, making it possible to recoup some of your expenses. Check with your local hospital or health unit for the possibility of receiving a subsidized rate for rental. Also, check with your health insurance company to see if the cost of a breast pump is covered under your policy. And finally, check with the Canada Customs and Revenue Agency, or your country's tax revenue department to see if you can claim a deduction for the breast pump as a medical expense (you will need a doctor's prescription for this).

Hospital-grade electric pumps are intended for multiple users and therefore have stronger motors. They also work on a closed system which ensures that milk droplets do not come in contact with the internal workings of the pump, thereby reducing or removing the risk of contamination for another user. Each new user uses their own pump kit (flanges and tubing). While this type of pump is not an absolute necessity, it is highly recommended- especially if you are a low volume producer, exclusively pumping from birth, or the mother of a premature baby.

It is a good idea to rent a hospital-grade pump for the first two or three months post-partum and then decide if you want to purchase a personal pump, such as the Pump In Style or the Purely Yours, or whether you wish to continue renting.

Hospital-grade electric pumps include such pumps as the Medela Lactina, Classic, and Symphony; and the Hollister/Ameda Elite, Lact-e, and SMB. The names of breast pumps may differ according to your location.

Other Types of Breast Pumps

Beyond the pumps already discussed, you will discover a couple others that are unique in their design. These pumps have very specific uses, and while some women may find success with them when exclusively pumping, they may not be the most appropriate choice and have not yet been proven to be effective to maintain a milk supply long-term.

The Whisper Wear pump is a very small pump which fits over the breast and can be worn under a shirt or bra. Two pumps must be used in order to double pump. Attached to the pump is a collection bag which hangs below. The benefit to this pump is that is operates very quietly and hands-free allowing the user to pump while doing other things.

This pump is relatively new and has undergone some revisions to improve its functioning. For the occasional user, it may be an interesting alternative, but it has not yet proven itself for exclusively pumping.

The other type of pump on the market that operates differently from the mainstream pumps is the Whittlestone Breast Expresser. This pump massages the nipple and areola with pulsating pads to encourage let-downs instead of relying on suction to remove milk. In fact, its suction level is very low compared to the suction levels of a baby at breast. This stimulation can be very good to initiate a supply and can work very well for women who want to start lactating for an adoptive baby, but it may not be as efficient in removing milk- and removal of milk is an absolute necessity to maintain your supply.

The Whittlestone Breast Expresser is reportedly very comfortable to use and stimulates a let-down very well; however, it has not yet proven itself as an effective pump for long-term exclusive pumping.

The Bottom Line

Without a doubt, the best pump to use when exclusively pumping is a hospital-grade double electric pump. These pumps not only have the durability to withstand constant use, they are also the most efficient pumps you can use to remove milk from your breasts. One obvious drawback of these pumps, though, is that they are not readily portable.

Consider renting a hospital-grade pump to initiate your milk supply. You can decide once your supply is established whether you want to purchase a pump or continue to rent. The use of a hospital-grade pump will give you the best start possible.

If you decide to purchase a pump, the majority of women exclusively pumping who use a personal pump use either the Medela Pump In Style or the Ameda Purely Yours. Both pumps will provide you with enough power while also allowing portability. You may also consider purchasing a slightly more expensive pump such as the Medela Lactina or Symphony or the Hollister/Ameda Elite which are still relatively lightweight and portable, yet a step above in terms of strength and reliability. The higher cost of purchasing this type of hospital-grade pump can be offset by the ability to sell it once you are finished pumping since they are intended as multiple-user pumps, and you may find that the cost of renting this type of pump long-term may be comparable to purchasing one.

Ultimately, the decision to rent or buy will depend on your individual situation and the length of time you plan on pumping. Obviously, the longer you pump the more sense it will make to purchase a pump of your own.

Individuality

As with many other things in life, different breast pumps will work for different women. Pumping should not be painful (provided you are not already suffering from thrush, cracked nipples, etc.). If you find one pump is causing pain, you feel it is not working effectively for you, or you just can't get consistent let-downs, try a different pump. (Ensure that you have first checked to see that you don't need a different sized flange or that you are not pumping at too high a suction level.) Switch manufacturers. Don't assume all pumps are the same; find one that works for you!

If you purchase a breast pump right from the start, the idea of switching to a different pump if you encounter problems may seem ludicrous. This is another reason why renting a pump at the beginning may be an excellent option. It will allow you to be sure your supply is well established, and also, it will allow you to test the type of pumps available.

Be sure to also look into whether your insurance company will pay for you to rent (or purchase) a breast pump, and remember, in many cases, you may be able to claim the cost of a breast pump as a medical expense on your income tax as long as you have a prescription from your doctor stating that it is medically necessary for your baby to have breast milk.

Accessories

Flanges

Flanges may also be referred to as horns or breast shields. The flange is the part of the pump that is placed over your breast and nipple and is attached to the tubing. The collection bottles are attached to the flanges. Flanges are usually made out of plastic, although there are some companies that offer softer silicone flanges or silicone inserts as well as extra large glass flanges.

Flanges can be purchased in different sizes allowing a woman to customize them to her particular needs. Ensure that the flange you use fits you well. Your nipples should not hit the end of the tube nor should they be squished into the flange. Some women find they require two different sized flanges. If you find that your nipples are hitting the end or feel that they are squished and you are experiencing discomfort, try a larger sized flange.

Medela offers the PersonalFit Breastshields. These shields are a two piece system that allows you to interchange the breast shield to meet your personal needs. The large shield is 27 mm in diameter and the extra large is 30 mm. They also carry an extra large glass breast shield to accommodate even larger nipples.

Ameda also offers a wide range of breast shield sizes to accommodate you. Their standard flange size is 25 mm. They also offer a custom flange that is 30.5 mm. With an insert, this custom flange is 28.5 mm in diameter. For smaller nipples, they offer a reducing insert for their standard flange reducing the size to 23 mm and further still to 21 mm if their Flexishield is used.

You may find the standard flange is too large for you. Often in this case, a large amount of the areola will be pulled into the flange tube causing excess friction on this part of the breast. If you find sores developing on your aerolas, ensure you are using a product such as lanolin to reduce the friction as much as possible. Also, try either smaller flanges, if they are available, or try a silicone insert such as the Ameda Flexishield or the Medela Softfit insert which will reduce the diameter of the flange while providing you with additional comfort.

Hands-free Pumping Bras

One of the negatives about exclusively pumping is sitting for up to 120 minutes a day pumping. But one of the positives about exclusively pumping is being able to sit for up to 120 minutes a day. The challenge, however, can be finding something to do while you are pumping that will allow you to relax, pass the time, and enjoy the time as your own. Reading, watching television, surfing the Internet, or catching up on email are all possible to do when pumping, and it can be nice to have this time for yourself. For some women though, trying to balance the flanges and bottles with only one hand while attempting to use the other can prove very difficult and frustrating. This is where a hands-free pumping bra can be of use.

There are a few different styles of pumping bras available from a few different manufacturers. Most hands-free pumping bras have slits in the front of the bra into which you slip the flange. One of the most common is the Easy Expression Hands-Free Bra which comes in two different styles: bustier or halter style bra. The bustier has a zip front and can easily be put on over a regular nursing bra before you pump. Made By Moms offers a pumping band. This product fits over a nursing bra and attaches around your chest using Velcro closures. Leading Lady manufactures a pumping bra that also doubles as a nursing bra. Medela offers nursing bras that can be used with their Pumping Free Attachment Kit. This bra and kit uses loops to attach your pump flange to the bra.

When deciding what kind of pumping bra you want to purchase, be sure you carefully consider how well they will stand up to the constant use. Consider the method the bra uses to hold the pump flanges. You do not want the bra to stretch and no longer hold the flanges tightly to your breast. You will also want it to be convenient, easy, and quick to use.

Another option is to make a pumping bra yourself. Some women simply take an old, snug fitting bra and cut slits into it for the flanges to fit in. You may find the holes you cut do stretch over time though, and this might be reason enough to purchase a bra designed especially for pumping.

While not a necessity for exclusively pumping, a hands-free pumping bra can allow you to use the time productively and allow you to pass the time without staring at your collection bottles. It may even allow you to enjoy your time pumping and use it as much deserved personal time.

Silicone Inserts

Ameda offers a silicone insert for the flange of their pump kit called the Ameda Flexishield. Medela offers the Softfit and Comfort Breastshield which are entirely made of silicone. The Medela shields must be used with the Medela Breastshield Connectors. These silicone inserts and flanges are intended to increase the comfort of the flanges while pumping as well as improve let-downs by increasing areola stimulation. The Ameda insert will also decrease the diameter of the flange which may be useful for women with small nipples.

Silicone inserts and flanges are not a necessary accessory for pumping. Many women do not use them and many women who have tried them did not find any benefit from them; some may even find them uncomfortable. However, in the right circumstance, these silicone accessories can make pumping much more comfortable and can increase the ease of let-downs.

If you are finding pumping continues to be uncomfortable for you, you are getting sores on your areolas caused by friction, or you are having difficulty consistently letting-down when pumping, then a silicone insert or flange may be worth trying.

Maintaining Your Pump, Pump Kit, and Collection System

It is important to collect and store breast milk as hygienically as possible. Maintaining your pump is the first step to ensuring your breast milk does not get contaminated.

Follow these guidelines in addition to the instructions provided with your pump:

- Wash your hands before handling your pump kit or using your pump.

- Wipe down your pump before and after each use.

- Cover your pump when not using it to protect it from dust and debris.

- Inspect the pump regularly for signs of wear or damage.

- Inspect the tubing regularly for signs of wear, punctures, condensation, or mold. Replace the tubing if necessary. Tubing may get condensation in it. If this happens, try running your pump with the tubing attached for a couple minutes to dry it out. If you notice mold in the tubing, replace it. With the open system pumps, you may discover milk has backed up into the tubing. While this is not common, it can happen. While you can rinse the tubing and hang it to dry, it is better to simply replace the tubing to ensure you are using parts that are as clean and uncontaminated as possible. The cost of additional tubing is minimal, especially when compared to the value of breast milk.

- The valves on the pump kit deserve special attention. Both the Medela and Ameda valves will wear and can tear. It is good preventative maintenance to replace them regularly- every three or four months. They are inexpensive and can make a difference in the effectiveness of your pump. Keep extra valves on hand in case the ones you are using tear.

- Dismantle your pump regularly and clean it thoroughly. Depending on the type of pump you are using, you will be able to dismantle it to varying degrees. Refer to the owner's manual or ask the rental station. If you are using the Pump In Style, be sure to remove the face plate regularly and clean behind it. Make it part of your routine to dismantle and clean your pump on a weekly basis. You will be amazed at how quickly dirt and grime can build up. Not only does this grime create a potential contamination risk for your milk, it can also decrease the efficiency of your pump creating a dangerous downward spiral of supply.

- Dismantle and clean your pump kit every time you pump. Since the pump kit is the part of the pump that the breast milk comes in direct contact with, it is vital that you keep it impeccably clean. Do not simply rinse the kit without taking it apart: remove all removable parts and wash each one in hot, soapy water. Rinse each part completely and allow to air dry. Once dry, either cover with a clean cloth to prevent contamination or place in a clean container or plastic storage bag.

- For ill or premature babies, pump kits should be sterilized after each use if you are pumping at the hospital. When at home, kits should be sterilized daily. It is good practice to sterilize your pump kit once a day even for full-term, healthy babies. Since you are storing breast milk for later use, it is best to prevent contamination of the breast milk whenever possible to allow for safe, long-term storage. If your own immunity has been compromised by a yeast infection, you *must* sterilize your equipment after each use.

- Some women who exclusively pump choose to simply rinse off their pump kit after using it, place it in a plastic storage bag, and store it in the refrigerator until the next pumping session. They choose to thoroughly clean their kit only once a day. This practice is based on the knowledge that expressed breast milk does not spoil at room temperature for several hours and will keep in the fridge for a number of days. This can certainly reduce the amount of time required for cleaning and make pumping, especially in the early months, more manageable. However, if you choose to do this, only do it if your baby is healthy and full-term. This practice does bring with it certain risks, and it is best if you clean your pump kit after each use.

- One way to make cleaning easier, especially if there no sink available for cleaning, is to use antibacterial cleansing cloths available from some pump manufacturers.

- Another option for simplifying your pumping routine and the amount of cleaning you need to do is to buy more than one pump kit. This will allow you to only wash your kits once or twice a day depending on how many kits you buy. If you are able to use a dishwasher to clean the kits, you will reduce your wash load quite dramatically.

- Sterilization of your pump kit should be done before its first use. You can sterilize in an open pot of boiling water or use a steam sterilizer. A steam sterilizer can be a very quick and time-conserving method to sterilize.

Since the breast pump you use is so extremely important to initiate and maintain your supply, take good care of it. Regular cleaning and maintenance will assist in not only ensuring the breast milk you collect remains free of contamination, but it will also ensure that the breast pump works as efficiently as possible for as long as possible. If you start to question whether the pump you are using is still working at its optimal level, do not hesitate to contact the manufacturer and speak to them about your concerns. You will find that most companies have exceptional customer service and will do whatever they can to see that you are able to continue pumping.

Using and Storing
Expressed Breast Milk

Proper storage and use of expressed breast milk is extremely important in order to provide your baby with the safest food possible. If you do your own research you will find that recommendations for the use and storage of expressed breast milk do vary; however, there are basic guidelines and ranges of storage times that are most commonly viewed as appropriate.

Learn the safe guidelines for using and storing expressed breast milk and practise them. Use your own best judgment. There is no point in working so hard to provide your baby with breast milk only to feed contaminated or soured milk or to have to discard expressed breast milk because it was not stored properly.

Collection Bottles

Just about any plastic or glass baby bottle will fit onto the major brands of breast pumps. The only exception is wide mouth bottles. However, you can purchase a conversion kit which will allow you to use Avent bottles with other pumps.

Pumping directly into feeding bottles can be especially useful if you are going to fed shortly after you pump since you can simply attach a nipple and feed without needing to transfer into another bottle or warm the milk. Your baby will also benefit the most from receiving freshly pumped milk. However, if you are going to store the expressed breast milk in the refrigerator, it is best to use collection bottles with tight fitting lids such as the ones that come with most breast pumps. You can also purchase these separately.

Ensure that collection bottles are carefully cleaned and preferably sterilized to ensure there is no contamination of your milk. Bottles must be sterilized for a pre-term or ill infant but may simply be washed in hot soapy water for full-term, healthy infants.

There are numerous places to purchase bottles to use for milk collection. Any department or drug store will sell common brands of baby bottles. Bottles made specifically for expressed milk can be purchased from any number of online stores selling breast pumps and accessories. Also, check with your local health unit and hospital to see if they sell pumps and accessories or if they can refer you to some place locally where you can purchase these supplies.

Another consideration when deciding on collection bottles is the size you wish to use. Most bottles made for expressed breast milk collection are four ounce bottles. Some baby bottles are four or five ounces, but many are eight or nine ounces in size. When your supply increases you may find you do sometimes need to switch bottles part way through a pumping session and you may therefore find that larger collection bottles are more convenient. In the beginning however, four ounce bottles should be adequate. Women with shorter torsos may find the larger bottles more cumbersome and difficult to handle due to their length.

Depending on your long-term storage requirements, use what works for you. There is no need to spend significant amounts of money on collection bottles, especially if you are not planning on using them to freeze or store long-term in your refrigerator.

Storage Containers for Fridge and Freezer Storage

It is important to carefully consider the containers you use to store your breast milk. Cost can become a factor if you are freezing large quantities though, and you may need to find a balance between the best storage containers and what you can afford. In general, choose the best, most protective containers you can afford.

There is some disagreement whether glass or plastic bottles are better for milk storage. The best depends on how you are storing the breast milk. Clear, hard plastic bottles made of polycarbonate that have tight fitting lids are the best choice for short-term storage in the refrigerator since leukocytes (white cells which fight infection) stick to glass. It is a good idea to invest in at least one set of breast milk storage bottles (the same ones can be used as collection bottles) for short-term storage in the refrigerator. For freezing, glass (brown glass being the absolute best choice) is the better choice because it provides better protection in the freezer since it is less porous than plastic. Freezing kills the leukocytes anyways, so the fact that leukocytes stick to glass is not a concern when freezing breast milk in glass containers.

Glass bottles for freezing can be difficult to find. Plastic bottles are also an acceptable alternative. If you decide to freeze in glass bottles, you can use baby food jars or small mason jars. Both of these options can be cost effective if you have a supply on hand or know of someone who does. Be sure to sterilize the jars and lids before using them. Another benefit of glass jars is that they can easily be sterilized and reused.

When freezing expressed breast milk, it is best to freeze in small amounts to reduce the amount of breast milk wasted if the entire amount is not eaten or needed once it is thawed. However, if you have large amounts of breast milk to freeze, this may not always be an option due to the expense of storage containers.

The next option for storage is plastic storage bags specifically designed for expressed breast milk. Medela, Ameda, Gerber, Bailey Medical, Lansinoh, and Avent all make bags for breast milk storage. Benefits of breast milk storage bags compared to other freezer bags include:

- pre-sterilized
- made of thicker plastic to protect from freezer burn and odors in freezer
- some are multi-ply
- some are also lined with nylon to prevent fat from sticking to the sides of the bag
- many have a zipper-type seal which help to prevent leakage
- and some fit onto pump kits.

Not all breast milk storage bags are created equal, so do your own research to determine which one is best for you.

Storage bags have a couple benefits over using glass or plastic bottles:

- quicker to thaw
- freezing flat can make better use of valuable freezer space.

You will need to decide what system is best for you.

The other option for freezing expressed breast milk is to use other types of plastic bags: freezer bags or bottle liners. Freezer bags are better since they have a sealed closure that will prevent leaks better. Bottle liners should be doubled to provide a stronger barrier and must be closed using twist ties which can easily lead to leakage or spillage of milk. With either type of bag, store several smaller bags inside a larger freezer bag to help prevent leaks and provide an extra barrier to protect the milk in the freezer.

Both bottle liners and freezer bags are not as good an option as other storage methods since they will cause antibodies and fat to adhere to the sides of the bags diminishing the benefits to your baby. They are, however, the most cost effective. If you plan on feeding frozen milk for any great length of time, consider investing in a more preferred option such as breast milk storage bags or glass or hard plastic bottles. But, if you can not afford the other options (and let's face it, it can get extremely expensive) then freezer bags are the better of these two.

Feeding Bottles

If you will not be breastfeeding at all, then use any bottle and nipple your baby likes. You may prefer to use a silicone nipple since they last longer and are easier to clean. You may also consider using an orthodontic type nipple.

If you are continuing to work on establishing breastfeeding or wanting to breastfeed for comfort, then you may want to use a wide-mouth bottle and nipple. Using a slow flow nipple will also continue to make your baby work for her milk and not get her used to the fast, easy flow of faster nipples.

If your baby suffers from severe colic or reflux, you may want to use a bottle that can reduce these symptoms.

Pumping and Storing Expressed Breast Milk

It is best to feed freshly expressed breast milk whenever possible since it maintains the largest amount of benefit for your baby. Refrigerated milk is second best and frozen milk is the next best.

If necessary, you can pump directly into previously pumped and cooled expressed breast milk as long as the cooled breast milk is no more than twenty-four hours old. Storage times are determined by the oldest milk. You can also pump directly into previously expressed milk that has been stored at room temperature as long as it is less than eight hours old (this depends on the room temperature). You must then, however, use this milk right away. You can also add chilled milk to previously frozen milk provided the amount you are adding is less than the amount frozen.

Be sure to always keep track of the date and time you express breast milk. Label all containers.

General Guidelines for Freezing Breast Milk

- Freeze in small amounts (two to four ounces) when possible.

- Milk expands when frozen, so ensure you leave sufficient room in the container to allow for expansion-about an inch should be enough.

- Write the date and amount of expressed breast milk on each storage container.

- There is some concern with using permanent marker on plastic bags due to the possibility of the marker leaching into the milk. Some bags avoid this concern by placing the labeling area outside of the storage chamber. To avoid this problem with other bags, use self-adhesive labels.

- Freeze bags of milk flat. After frozen, you may stack them or, better yet, place a number of bags into a larger freezer bag for storage.

- Reorganize your expressed breast milk in the freezer often, keeping the newest milk at the bottom or back of the freezer and bringing the oldest milk to the top or the front. Be sure to always use the oldest milk first.

- Check your freezer regularly to ensure it is operating properly. Be sure everyone in your family understands how important it is to keep the freezer door closed.

- If you are storing expressed breast milk in a fridge at work or in someone else's home, it is best to label it as expressed breast milk.

Storage Times

Below is a chart showing the range of storage times for breast milk dependent upon the type of storage. These are guidelines and your judgment should also be used, taking into consideration your baby's needs and the environmental temperature. Also, these are the *maximum* recommended storage times. It is best to always use expressed breast milk as soon as possible, refrigerate it as soon as possible, and freeze it if it will not be used within twenty-four to forty-eight hours.

Also, it is quite possible that under the right conditions, breast milk can be stored for longer than six months in a deep freezer with some sources suggesting up to a year. It is best not to extend the storage times within a refrigerator or refrigerator freezer though, since the temperature of these appliances does not remain consistent due to frequent opening of the door.

It is also important to always maintain your storage containers and pump equipment as well as possible, thoroughly cleaning them in order to store your expressed breast milk as long as possible without any concern of contamination or spoilage.

Type of Storage	Storage Temperature	Recommended Maximum Storage Times*
Room Temperature	15°C 60°F	up to 24 hours
	19-22°C 66-72°F	up to 10 hours
	25°C 79°F	up to 4-6 hours
Refrigerator	0-4°C 32-39°F	up to 8 days
	4-10°C 39-50°F	up to 3 days
Freezer Compartment inside of refrigerator	variable temperature due to frequent door opening	2 weeks
Freezer Separate door as part of refrigerator	variable temperature due to frequent door opening	3-4 months
Separate Chest-Type Deep Freeze	-19°C 0°F	6 months +

* There is a very limited amount of research on safe storage times for expressed breast milk. It is best to always use breast milk as quickly as possible, refrigerate as soon as possible, or freeze within twenty-four to forty-eight hours.

Using Fresh Milk

- It is best to use fresh breast milk as much as possible since there is less deterioration of its elements. However, it is best to refrigerate expressed breast milk as soon as possible. In order to accommodate both recommendations, leave out only enough breast milk for your baby's next feeding and refrigerate or freeze the rest.

- Research has shown that expressed breast milk can be safely kept at room temperature for up to eight or ten hours. However, it is the caveat "up to" that must be heeded. It may last that long, but it may not. Much depends on the conditions in which it is kept.

- Always smell and taste the milk before feeding to be sure it has not soured, especially if it has sat out for awhile. Usually smelling it will be enough to determine if it is okay, but if it is in question, taste it as well. Some people may be turned off by the thought of tasting breast milk, but it really is the best way to determine if there is any concern with it.

- Freshly pumped milk can make going out on a trip to the grocery store, the park, or out to lunch much easier since you will not need to worry about cooling the milk as long as you will be using it within a couple hours. You will also not need to warm the milk since it will be kept at room temperature.

Using Refrigerated Milk

- Always use the oldest expressed breast milk first.

- There is a very limited amount of research that shows breast milk can be refrigerated for up to eight days at 0-4°C (32-39°F). However, safe food practices recommend freezing any milk that is not used within twenty-four to forty-eight hours. If you are pumping more than your baby requires, it is good practice to freeze any excess breast milk on a daily basis.

- Smell and taste the milk before feeding to ensure it has not soured.

- You can warm the milk, although some people choose not to. It can be gentler on little tummies to warm the milk and assist in warding off colic symptoms.

- Gently swirl the milk to mix in any separated fat. Do not shake the milk! Shaking can break down the proteins in breast milk.

Using Frozen Milk

- Always use the oldest milk first to extend the life of your freezer stash.

- The best method to thaw breast milk is in the fridge. Depending on your storage container, this can take anywhere from twelve to twenty-four hours.

- You can also place the frozen milk in a container of warm water or run under cool water until thawed.

- If you use heat to thaw milk, you must use it right away.

- Once thawed, breast milk can be kept in the refrigerator for up to twenty-four hours.

- Thawed breast milk is much more fragile and you may find it deteriorates quickly. It may not last twenty-four hours after thawing.

- Do not refreeze thawed milk.

- Once milk has been warmed, it must be used within one hour or discarded.

Warming Expressed Breast Milk

To warm cold breast milk, you can place it in a container of warm water until it reaches room temperature or slightly warmer. You can also use a bottle warmer. Do not use boiling water.

Never heat breast milk on the stove or in a microwave. Not only can this cause hot spots in the milk that can scald the baby, but it can also destroy vital properties in the milk. Always test the temperature of the milk after gently mixing it and before feeding it to your baby.

Feeding Expressed Breast Milk

- Use the feeding bottle of your choice.

- Feed on cue instead of by a schedule.

- Feed as much as your baby wants. Learn your baby's cues as to when he is hungry and when he has had enough.

- Do not encourage your baby to finish every bottle if he seems like he has had enough. Breastfeeding reduces the incidence of obesity. This may be a factor of breast milk itself; however, it may be due to the baby's ability to self-regulate his intake when at the breast. For this reason, allow your baby to determine how much milk he needs.

- Babies have an intrinsic need to suck. It may not be possible for a baby to satisfy this need by bottle feeding alone. Consider using a pacifier in order to meet this need. Some babies will overeat simply to satisfy their need to suck. If your baby is noticeably uncomfortable after eating large amounts or spitting up large amounts of milk, offer a pacifier and see if this will satisfy him.

- A very rough formula to determine milk intake in the early days and weeks is weight in pounds X 2.5= daily intake in ounces. This is used for formula feeding as well and doesn't take into consideration the variation between individuals' breast milk composition. A number of studies have shown that a breastfeeding mother's milk production does not significantly change between one and six months post-partum, so the belief that a baby's intake should increase as they gain weight may very well be a misconception.

- Average maximum intake will be around 900-960 milliliters (30-32 ounces) per day.

- Intake will slowly decline after the introduction of solids as solid meals start to replace the required calories.

Unused Expressed Breast Milk after a Feeding

If your baby does not finish the expressed breast milk offered during a feeding, consider the following:

- It is best to discard any breast milk remaining in the bottle after a feeding. However, some sources suggest that it is okay to refrigerate this milk if it is used within a couple hours for the next feeding. If you choose to do this, do not do it with milk that has been frozen and it is best to do it only with fresh milk as opposed to milk that has been stored in the refrigerator.

- If the milk was previously refrigerated or frozen, dump any milk that is remaining after the feeding.

- Do not reheat milk that has been previously heated.

Once again, use your judgment and err on the side of caution.

The Look and Smell of Expressed Breast Milk

Fresh

Breast milk may have a slightly bluish colouration. The colour of breast milk can change depending on the mother's diet or medication she may take. Breast milk is rather thin, but this does not have a direct relationship to the fat content of the milk. It usually has no noticeable smell and has a slightly sweet taste.

Refrigerated

Breast milk that has been stored in the refrigerator has the same colour and taste as fresh milk. It will separate with a layer of fatty cream forming at the top. The fat may also form into clumps. The fat can be gently mixed into the milk before being fed to the baby. Expressed breast milk can take on the smells of other foods in the fridge. Use a box of baking soda to limit this. Also, use quality storage containers and avoid keeping strong smelling foods such as onions in the fridge.

For those women with very high lipase levels, expressed breast milk may, after sitting for a while, begin to smell like vomit. Lipase aids the baby in breaking down the fat in the breast milk, and this smell is a result of it doing its job. In effect, the milk is being digested. As long as the milk is not sour, it is okay to feed. Most babies will not notice the smell. If your baby does not accept the milk, you may need to take some extra steps to preserve your breast milk.

To limit the effects of the lipase, you can scald your breast milk briefly on the stove prior to storing it. Heat it on a low heat just until small bubbles break the surface, but do not boil the milk.

Frozen

After thawing, breast milk will be the same colour as fresh or refrigerated breast milk. Some slight variation is possible. The smell and taste of frozen milk can be altered from freezing. Often, women report a soapy or metallic smell to thawed breast milk. The taste may also reflect the smell. It can also smell like vomit due to the activity of lipase. Generally, if your baby accepts the milk, it is fine to use. If your baby refuses it, however, you may need to make some changes. You may consider the following:

- Try freezing breast milk in a different type of container.

- Avoid the use of a self-defrosting freezer if possible since the thaw/freeze of the defrost cycle may affect the breast milk. If this is not possible, try not to store the breast milk next to the walls of the freezer.

- Change your thawing method.

- Reduce the length of time you are storing the milk after thawing it. Thawed breast milk is very fragile and deteriorates quickly.

- Scald your milk before freezing it.

- Cool your milk before freezing it, or freeze it directly after being pumped.

If breast milk has gone bad, it will smell and taste sour. If you are ever in doubt, it is best to discard it. Use your judgment, but remember it is always best to err on the side of caution.

Freezer Failure/Power Outages

Unfortunately, power outages and freezer failures are a possibility. It is best to be prepared and have a plan in place to either guard against these situations or know how to deal with them if they do arise.

Be sure to check your freezer often to ensure it is operating properly. If you find that it has failed, check all of the milk immediately. Any that is still frozen should be put into a cooler with ice or freezer packs and transferred to a working freezer as soon as possible. You can also use as much as possible within the next twenty-four to thirty-six hours depending how long ago your freezer failed. Never refreeze thawed breast milk.

If you have a power outage, cover your freezer with blankets to add to the insulation and keep the cold in. Do not open the freezer unless absolutely necessary. The contents of the freezer should stay frozen for at least forty-eight hours if it is full (always keep your freezer as full as possible- it will also work more efficiently this way). Once power has been restored, check the frozen milk carefully. The milk stored on the outside of the freezer is most vulnerable.

Lack of Storage Space

If you are freezing large amounts of breast milk, you may find that your freezer space soon disappears. Consider buying a larger freezer. Compared to the cost of formula, the added expense of buying a freezer may not seem so costly. A stand-up model is easier to fill and makes it easier to rotate the frozen milk.

Donate to a Milk Bank

For those women blessed with a more than ample supply and limited freezer space, the question that eventually arises is, "What do I do with all this milk?" In some situations, donating your milk may be the answer. Prematurity, adoption, and maternal death or illness are examples of why human breast milk may be required from a donated source.

In Canada, the only milk bank currently operating is at the Children's and Women's Health Care Centre in Vancouver, British Columbia. Donating to this milk bank may prove difficult due to your location and transportation issues. However, by contacting other organizations in your community such as La Leche League or the local health unit, you may be able to find a need right in your own community.

In the United States, milk banks are more plentiful. Milk banks are located in California, Texas, North Carolina, Iowa, Delaware, and Colorado (see "Resources" for the web site address for the Human Milk Banking Association of North America). However, due to limited resources, both financial and physical, milk banks may not always be able to accept donations. Contact the closest milk bank to you to check their donation status, and if they are not accepting at that time, widen your search from there. Some banks will pay for expenses associated with storage and shipping.

There are also milk banks in numerous other countries throughout the world. Check to see whether donating to a milk bank is possible where you live.

Donations are usually a minimum of 3 liters or 100 ounces. When donating your milk, your health will be thoroughly checked and blood testing will be required to screen for various illnesses. It is also important that you have not taken any medication or herbal supplements while pumping. There are a few exceptions to this such as insulin or pre-natal vitamins. Check with the milk bank for a list of exceptions. Ineligibility would also arise from other risks factors such as consumption of alcohol, cigarette smoking, being at high risk for HIV due to lifestyle or partner's HIV status or lifestyle, blood transfusion or organ transplant within six months of lactation, as well as certain travel restrictions.

Selling human milk is illegal whereas donating milk is a true act of kindness. By donating your milk, you will be helping another child receive the best start to life possible and impact that child into the future.

Traveling Long Distances with Frozen Milk

If you are moving or traveling and need to transport frozen breast milk, the best way to do this is to pack it in a cooler with dry ice and newspaper. Check your local yellow pages to find a supplier of dry ice.

On the Go with Expressed Breast Milk

Getting out of the house can sometimes seem like quite the challenge when you are pumping, but going out with expressed breast milk can actually be quite easy. If you pump just before you leave, you can take that fresh milk with you. It will be fine for a few hours depending on the temperature. Check the storage guidelines chart in this chapter.

If it is very hot out or the milk has been previously cooled, you can use a portable cooler bag with ice packs to keep the milk chilled. To warm the milk you have several options:

- Run it under hot tap water.
- Ask for a cup of warm water from a restaurant.
- Bring a thermos of hot water with you to warm the bottle.
- Warm the bottle between your hands or thighs to take the chill off it.
- Take the bottle of milk out of the cooler 10-15 minutes before feeding to allow it to warm up slightly.
- Feed the milk cold. Some babies will not mind the occasional cold bottle.

Overcoming Difficulties

In a previous chapter, some of the negative aspects of exclusively pumping were mentioned. Difficulties will almost inevitably arise, and overcoming them will sometimes require a great deal of resourcefulness, patience, acceptance, effort, and determination on your part. These difficulties fit into a wide range of categories; however, all of them can be enough to make you consider quitting. For many of the difficulties you encounter, as with many things in life, time will often resolve the problem; however, when you are in the middle of the situation, it is often difficult to remove yourself from the present and see things in perspective. Remember that you will be pumping for only a short time when you balance it out in terms of your life or your child's life. While it may not seem possible, time will pass and you will move with it. Each pumping session will take you closer to your goal. The first couple months of your new baby's life will move at a snail's pace and every problem you encounter will be magnified as you try to get accustomed to your new life. With any difficulty you encounter, recognize that it will often pass with time and that things will soon settle into a comfortable routine. No obstacle in insurmountable, yet some require a little extra time and effort.

Lack of Sleep

Lack of sleep is certainly not unique to the life of a mom who is pumping exclusively; however, due to the extra time involved to pump and then bottle feed, there seems to be fewer hours in a day for pumping moms. The old adage, "sleep when your baby sleeps", is often unrealistic if you are exclusively pumping since the time when your baby sleeps is a prime pumping opportunity. In order to build a strong supply, it is important to pump in the night at least once, which means your night feeds become an hour or more in length.

So how do you get sleep? Well, in some ways, resign yourself to the fact that you will be sleep deprived. But there are a few things you may consider:

- Enlist the help of anyone you can get to help. If someone offers to take the baby while you pump, let them. If someone offers to cook dinner, let them. If someone offers to get you some groceries, let them.

- Talk to your friends and family about what you are doing. Explain to them the importance of breast milk for your baby. Explain how important it is to you that your baby is fed breast milk. Once people understand what you are doing and the reasons you are doing it, they will likely be more inclined to offer help and limit the expectations they place on you.

- Sleep when you can and don't worry about the house.

- Keep good sleep habits when possible. Try to keep some sort of regular bedtime schedule (as difficult as that may be). Try not to eat too late into the evening. Keep your bedroom conducive to sleep: draw the curtains, use soft light, and don't use the space to watch television or pay your bills.

- Let your partner take the night feeds occasionally or do the last evening feeding and put the baby to bed so that you can go to bed early. Even if you only do this once in a while, it will make you feel much better. Unfortunately, we can't stockpile our hours of sleep, so getting in a good night's sleep every once in a while will keep you sane.

- Remember that all moms are facing sleep deprivation, too. It will get better!

Sore Nipples and Breast Pain

Not all women who exclusively pump will be faced with nipple soreness. However, it is a possibility and one that can lead you to consider quitting. This is not necessary. It is important to understand the many reasons that you may be facing soreness and head the problem off before it begins if possible, or at least resolve the problem as quickly as possible.

The following are some common reasons you may experience soreness when pumping:

Yeast Infection

Yeast infections, or thrush, are fairly common in breastfeeding women. A yeast infection is characterized by a burning pain, deep tissue pain if the yeast is also in the breast ducts, redness and shininess of the nipple, itchiness, and the possibility of yeast infection in your baby's mouth or diaper area. Receiving antibiotics during labour can increase the chances of a yeast overgrowth as can a general tendency towards yeast infections.

Yeast can be transferred between mother and baby if exclusively pumping through the breast milk, and if breastfeeding, it can be transferred from baby to mother through contact with the nipple. If you suspect your baby may have thrush, look for white patches in your baby's mouth that do not wash off. Soreness and redness in the mouth and throat caused by the yeast can sometimes cause the baby to refuse to eat. In the diaper area, yeast will show as a red diaper rash, usually in small circles or spots and will show no improvement with the use of a diaper cream. If you think your baby has thrush, see your baby's doctor to receive treatment. Many doctors will recommend a baby be treated for thrush if the mother has been diagnosed with it and the baby is being breastfed.

If you develop what you think is a yeast infection, see your doctor as soon as possible and start treatment. Gentian violet is a good first course of action that is relatively effective and inexpensive. Depending on the severity of the infection, you may need to start on oral medications as well. It is important to realize that yeast overgrowth is a systemic problem and must be viewed as such. Therefore, try to cut out your intake of sugars and simple carbohydrates as well as improve your intestinal flora by taking acidophilus supplements. A healthy diet, strong immune system, and healthy digestive tract are vital to keeping a yeast overgrowth at bay.

It is also important to prevent re-infecting yourself with the materials that come in contact with your breasts. Yeast is particularly resilient and it may take some effort to rid your system of the overgrowth. Be sure to:

- Change your breast pads frequently if you are using them.
- Wash your bras daily in hot water.
- Wash your bath towel after every use in hot water.
- Sterilize your pump kit after every use.
- Sterilize your collection bottles.
- Sterilize your baby's feeding bottles.
- Do not use lanolin as a lubricant since it will keep your nipples moist which can encourage yeast growth.

If you are breastfeeding in addition to pumping, your doctor may recommend treating your baby for thrush as well even if he is not showing signs of the infection.

Dr. Jack Newman's articles are an excellent source of information on yeast overgrowth and treatments. You can find them at www.breastfeedingonline.com. Another informative site for information about the treatment of thrush is www.kellymom.com.

Blocked Ducts

A blockage in a milk duct can occur when lactating. Many women will experience a block. Pumping may make you more susceptible to blocked ducts since one of the causes can be the failure to empty your breasts sufficiently. Some women will find they are highly prone to blocked ducts, and, if this is the case, you will want to take this into consideration when dropping pumps or weaning.

Symptoms of a blocked duct include soreness or pain in a localized area of your breast, redness around the area, a hard lump that can vary in size depending on how large the blockage is, and a decrease in milk volume.

It is extremely important to resolve a block as soon as possible since it can lead to mastitis if not dealt with. Try to avoid blocked ducts by removing as much milk as possible from your breasts as often as possible. Do not make sudden or drastic alterations to your pumping schedule, and do not wear tight, restrictive bras or underwire bras.

Treatment for blocked ducts:

- Pump! Pump often and longer if necessary to work out the blockage.

- Massage the affected area prior to and while pumping.

- Use breast compressions while pumping. Do not be overly forceful, however, since you can damage breast tissue.

- Use heat on the affected area. Take a hot shower before pumping or use a warm compress on the site. One pumping mom reported good success using heat patches for sore muscles that are available in the drug store.

- If there is a blister on the nipple, you may need to lance it with a sterile needle in order to free the blockage.

- In stubborn cases, ultrasound may work to break up the blockage.

- Lecithin capsules also benefit some women. These may be worth considering if you are prone to blocked ducts. See Kellymom.com for the recommended dosage of lecithin.

Mastitis

Mastitis is an infection of the breast. It can arise from a blocked duct if left untreated, but this is not always the case. Symptoms are similar to a blocked duct but are usually more severe in terms of pain, inflammation, and redness. Mastitis is also often accompanied by a fever and overall sense of being unwell.

Treatment for mastitis:

- Mastitis requires a physician's intervention and treatment as soon as possible.

- Antibiotics are usually required and will be prescribed by your doctor.

- Do not stop pumping since engorgement will worsen the symptoms and can result in blocked ducts which will worsen the situation.

- Check with your doctor to ensure the medication being prescribed is compatible with breastfeeding.

- Rest as much as possible.

- Use heat on the area of infection.

- Use ibuprofen for pain and inflammation or acetaminophen for pain.

Using too high a suction level on your pump

Using too high a suction level is one of the major causes of nipple trauma when pumping. Many women find that when they turn down the suction they actually increase their yield since it is more comfortable and often will increase let-downs. Find the minimum suction level that will work for you. Some pumps will actually produce enough suction to seriously damage your breast! Don't trust that the pump is calibrated in such a way that the highest suction will work the best or even be safe.

Friction

Friction is a problem that can be easily avoided, but one that is not often mentioned to women who are pumping. The friction caused by the pump can definitely cause pain and soreness. The best line of defense is to use a lubricating product such as lanolin before you pump. Lanolin is contraindicated if you are suffering from a yeast infection. Olive oil is recommended by some lactation consultants and may offer some antibacterial properties as well.

Another source of pain caused by friction can be flanges that are too small. If you have large nipples and find that your nipples are rubbing against the sides of the flanges when you are pumping, you may want to try a larger flange.

Conversely, flanges that are too large and that allow a large amount of the areola to be pulled into the flange when pumping can also cause pain and discomfort. If this is the case you can try a smaller flange, if available, or try a soft silicone insert that will reduce the diameter of the flange.

The Pump

There are a number of pumps on the market. Pumps are different. The suck and release cycles will vary by pump and manufacturer. If you have tried to remedy pain caused by pumping and have not found any success, consider trying a different pump. I attempted to switch pumps half-way through my year of pumping. I switched from one of the major brands to the other, and I lasted for only two pumping sessions! I found the new pump so extremely painful that there was no way I could even consider using it. I promptly returned to my original pump and finished the year with it.

There are other causes of pain during pumping such as Reynauld's phenomenon, eczema, and other skin sensitivities. These, however, are best dealt with at your doctor's office.

In general, take good care of your breasts and nipples! Here are some general guidelines for breast care:

- Don't use soap on your breasts when bathing.
- Change your breast pads regularly.
- Wash your clothes with a mild, fragrance free detergent.
- Wash your bras regularly.
- Allow your nipples to air dry when possible.

- Leave some breast milk on your nipples after pumping to assist in warding off infections and to help prevent dryness.

Responding to People Who Ask If You Are Breastfeeding

Invariably, someone will ask you if you are breastfeeding and often women who exclusively pump are uneasy or unsure of how to answer. It really is up to you. I would suggest you have two equally appropriate options:

- Answer "yes". This is probably the easiest and quickest answer; however, it may lead to quizzical looks when you pull out a bottle to feed your baby. But it is true- you are "breastfeeding by bottle".

- Accept any opportunity to tell people about the option of exclusively pumping and the fact that is a viable alternative to formula feeding.

Your decision on how to handle this question is often determined by who it is asking the question. In general though, it is a positive thing to explain how beneficial breast milk is to an infant and how you have dedicated yourself to providing breast milk for your child.

Feelings of Resentment Toward Your Pump

Yes, it is true, you will, at some point in time, resent your pump. You will look at it as though it is a living, breathing creature that has pushed its way into your life to destroy every spare moment you once had. You will often feel attached to your pump- physically attached to it that is. You may even go so far as to cover it up with a large blanket so you don't have to look at it. This, I'm afraid, is all part of the decision to exclusively pump.

When pregnant, I imagined what it would be like to leave the hospital with my newborn and take him home. However, when he was born at thirty-one weeks gestation things did not work out as planned. When I was released from the hospital three days after his birth, he did not come with me. Instead of leaving with my baby, I left with a breast pump. And the breast pump stayed with me for the next year. We (the pump and I that is) had a kind of love-hate relationship. There were times when I hated the sight of it and the resignation I felt knowing that I needed to hook up to it instead of being able to go to bed. But I also loved the fact that it enabled me to nourish my son for the first year of his life.

The best advice I can give when you are feeling tied to your pump is to take it one pump at a time. Don't think about the long-term, but think only of the present. Consider what this contraption is allowing you to do and what it is providing for your child. There was a time when exclusively pumping was not an option since the breast pumps available were not nearly effective enough to initiate or maintain a milk supply. Be thankful that we are able to access to this technology.

Another suggestion that might help is to become portable. Using a personal pump such as the Medela Pump In Style or Ameda Purely Yours can allow you to pump on the go. This kind of pump allows you to pump pretty much anywhere- even when in the car. If you are comfortable with this, it is a definite solution to being tied down at home because you have to pump.

And as was said before, it does get easier. Early on, you have to pump so often that leaving the house can become a very onerous task. By the time you pump, pack up, get your baby ready and yourself ready, it is almost time to pump again and leaving the house hardly seems worth it. But this won't last for long. As you start dropping pumps, you will gain more time away from your pump, and you will gain the freedom you require.

Juggling a Baby and a Pumping Schedule

Early on in your newborn's life, pumping will not be as difficult to fit in as it will become in a couple months. Although you will have to pump often, hopefully your baby will be sleeping most of the day away with only brief alert periods and you will be able to pump while your baby is sleeping. Unfortunately, this makes it impossible to follow that ever constant advice to sleep while your baby is sleeping. If you're lucky, you might be able to get a few minutes in before your baby needs you again.

Once your baby gets a few months under his belt, pumping will be a little easier since you will now be able to entertain your child with various devices and contraptions such as a bouncy chair, a baby video, an exersaucer, or a swing. Pumping that can not be done during nap times can often be done while your baby entertains himself with one of these activities.

It is the months in between the newborn stage and the stage when your baby can finally entertain himself for a while that will pose the greatest challenge to your pumping. From about two months to three or four months, your baby will be awake for longer periods, perhaps be more resistant to napping, and require your interaction constantly to fill in the awake time. This can be stressful and exasperating when you want to pump but your baby's schedule will not work with yours.

First, know that this period will pass and, in most cases, you will soon have a child who is able to be alone for short periods without too much trouble. You will also be able to drop pumps soon which will allow you to stretch out the time between pumping sessions if needed. As well, it is important to understand that the number of pumping sessions in a day is probably more important than the length of time between sessions. If you are trying to fit six sessions into a day, don't worry about spacing them all exactly four hours apart. If, for example, you have pumped two hours ago and your baby falls asleep in the car on the way home and continues sleeping when you bring him in, then use this unexpected nap time to pump! Chances are you will have more difficulty doing it later once your little one wakes up. You will most likely find that the pumping session after only two hours has a slightly reduced yield, but the next pump (which will likely be after four or five hours) will produce a greater volume. In the end, all will usually even itself out.

Of course, another thing you must do is to accept help when it is offered. It can be difficult enough just taking care of a new baby, but adding in the pumping can make it seem unmanageable. Take people up on their offers to help out. Have a honest discussion with your spouse and share with him the importance to you of providing breast milk for your baby- he will probably share in your desire to feed your baby breast milk. Share your emotions and your needs with him so he can understand what you are going through. Share with him the ways in which he can support you in your decision to exclusively pump. The time you are pumping is a great opportunity for dad to get some one-on-one time with his new baby!

Most of all, recognize that you are not going to do this alone. Even if the help you receive is simply moral and emotional support, it will make a world of difference. A shoulder to cry on and a strong arm to pull you back up when you feel you can't continue will make a world of difference in trying to exclusively pump for the long haul.

Overwhelming Desires to Quit

If you never have this overwhelming desire to quit pumping, then I would suggest you're not human! Exclusively pumping is taxing- both mentally and physically. You are doing double duty when it comes to feeding your baby and it will take its toll on you. Fortunately, the good days usually outnumber the bad days.

When one of these horrible days strike, first consider the reasons you are pumping. Often, simply remembering that you are doing this for the health and future of your child will be enough to get you through. For some women, the financial cost of switching to formula will also play into why they are choosing to pump. And sometimes, it will simply be personal accomplishment that will keep you pumping.

One of the most important elements of successful pumping is building and using a support system. This may come from the Internet, friends or family, a doctor or lactation consultant, or any other person you can go to for support. Ideally, this person will have some experience with exclusively pumping or breastfeeding and have knowledge about pumping. Use your support system. It is one of the biggest indicators of success with exclusively pumping. The desire to quit is often frustration with a particular situation instead of a genuine desire to wean.

Everyone will get to a point, though, when the thought of weaning starts entering their mind. It is at this point when you have to carefully survey the situation. Consider the following:

- Is the reason for considering weaning because of a certain situation or event in your life which will change or pass? If there is something specific causing you to consider weaning, perhaps you could/should wait until it passes in order to make a clear-headed decision. Try not to make a rash decision about weaning without considering the whole picture.

- How close are you to your long-term goal? Perhaps you have already passed your long-term goal. Perhaps you are close enough to it that, through a long weaning process, you will still meet it. Perhaps you will realize that your goal needs to be adjusted or that it is not as important as you once thought it was. Or perhaps you will recognize that you really want to achieve your goal.

- How will you feel if you decide to wean now? A certain amount of guilt over weaning is to be expected, but it should not consume you. Will you feel proud of yourself for pumping as long as you did? Or will you feel like you failed and didn't try hard enough? If possible, try to keep pumping long enough to work through these emotions ahead of time.

- How much breast milk do you have in your freezer? Women with extremely large stashes in their freezer can feed breast milk for two months or more after they wean. This can allow you to wean a couple months ahead of your goal if you so desire and still meet your goal.

- Is your baby over six months of age? Passive immunity usually ends around six months. If your reasons for feeding breast milk to your baby centre around this particular immunological benefit, then six months is a great goal. Of course, remember that the immunological benefits of breast milk are just a small part of the benefits a baby derives from mother's milk.

- How much support do you have for exclusively pumping? Without a strong support system, it can be difficult to handle the daily pressures of pumping. You will need to look into yourself and determine if you are able to continue on your own and if the benefits to your child are worth your stress and other difficulties that you are facing. Weigh it carefully. Your child benefits from your milk, but he also benefits from a healthy and happy mommy.

- Do you feel as though you could continue if you had to? Often, we feel as though we simply can not continue on, but this is rarely the case. Look deep into yourself; ask yourself the tough questions. Draw on your reserves. If you do not have any reserves to draw on, then perhaps it is time to wean.

- Are you currently able to meet your baby's daily intake requirements? If you are a low volume producer and are not meeting your baby's daily intake, you may get to a point where you ask yourself if it is worth it. As always, only you can answer this. Any amount of breast milk will benefit your baby. However, if you are fighting to maintain your supply and feel you are losing the battle, you should allow yourself to consider how much more you would be able to give your baby if you were not pumping. Does it balance out or would not pumping provide more?

You will have days when you are simply having a hard time pumping and you hate the idea of having to "hook up" to the pump yet again. During these times, the best thing to do is to simply go one pump at a time. Don't think about the long-term. Usually you will find that these feelings pass: your baby starts napping well and you have time to pump, or your mother visits for a week and is able to play with the baby while you pump. Often by taking it one pump at a time, one day at a time, you will discover that you can do this much longer than you ever thought possible.

Building and Maintaining Relationships While Exclusively Pumping

Motherhood brings about many changes. Changes in your relationships with family, friends, spouse, and older children are almost inevitable. Often this change is good and builds a deeper, stronger relationship. But sometimes, arriving at that stronger relationship can be a trying and often stressful experience.

If you add exclusively pumping into the mix, you may find that your relationships are even more difficult to maintain. It is important to be open with your family and friends and allow them to understand your decision to pump. Recognize that not only is this something that you personally need to deal with, but also something that your family and friends may need to adjust to.

This chapter will offer some suggestions for building a relationship with your new baby while maintaining a strong relationship with your older children, family, friends, and spouse. The suggestions are by no means an exhaustive list but will perhaps start you thinking about how your entire support circle is affected by your decision to exclusively pump and ways in which they can learn to support you while still receiving the attention from you that they require.

Building a Strong Bond with Your New Baby

Unfortunately, some women who exclusively pump are told by others that they are doing their baby a disservice by not breastfeeding and that they will not build a strong bond with their baby because of it. While breastfeeding does provide an excellent bonding relationship, it is by no means the only way a mother and baby bond. The following are some suggestions for building a strong bond with your new baby:

- Make time for your baby. Leave other things such as the dishes or vacuuming undone when possible. Allow yourself to spend one-on-one time with your baby.

- Lots of skin-to-skin contact with your baby, especially in the early days, can help to establish a strong bond and will also aid in milk production. Take a break in the afternoon and lay down with your baby on your chest. Not only will you enjoy the closeness, but your baby will also benefit from your warmth and the connection he will have to your breathing.

- Do not bottle prop. Turn off the television when feeding your baby. Use the time to gaze at him, sing, talk, smile, laugh...

- Consider wearing your baby in a sling or other type of carrier. Wearing your baby not only frees you up to do other things while still meeting the needs of your child, it also meets your baby's need for physical contact, security, stimulation, and movement. Babies worn in a sling often cry less than babies not worn. The baby's close proximity to you will also assist in maintaining body temperature and regulating respiration and heart rate.

- Pumping hands free can allow you to play with your baby while pumping. Using a hands free pumping bra will give you the freedom to sit on the floor, read a book to your baby, or play with your baby.

- Recognize that you are providing nourishment for your baby. While it may take some time away from her, it is providing a lot as well. It is a balancing act that will take you a little time to get used to.

Your Relationship With Other Children

A new baby can be a huge adjustment for children you may already have. Often there is a period of jealousy or anger at losing out on the status he or she might have enjoyed. Suddenly, there is a new baby that must fit into their world. You will no doubt have considered ways to make this adjustment easier on your other children.

When you start to exclusively pump, you are now adding another element of change into your child's life. You may not have as much time to spend with her and you may find that you are more house-bound for a few weeks when you are frequently pumping. Your child may start to resent your pumping. Here are a few ideas to help older children adjust to all the new things happening in your home and ways to maintain a strong relationship with them while you are pumping:

- Depending on their age, explain to them what you are doing and why you are doing it. Use language that they can understand and don't get too technical. Explain that mommy's milk is the best food for babies and you need to pump to provide the baby milk.

- Explain how you fed them and why you are feeding the new baby this way.

- Allow them to be part of the routine. Give them special tasks such as turning on the pump, bringing you things you might need while you are pumping, or playing with the baby while you pump. Let them be an important element of the success.

- Consider your time pumping as an opportunity to spend time with older children. For example, if your baby is sleeping and doesn't require your attention when you pump give this time to your older child: read a story, sing songs, or play games such as "I Spy" or "Simone Says" which don't require too much participation on your part.

- Most importantly, don't consider your older children another obstacle to pumping.

- If your older child is still quite young and unable to understand what you are doing or unable to be on his own while you pump, recognize that he may see the pump and the new baby as something that has taken his mother away. Be prepared to spend some one-on-one time with your other child and recognize that new behaviours may simply be a reaction to this change. Be patient and understanding.

Maintaining Your Relationship with Friends and Family

Hopefully, most of your friends and family will be supportive of your decision to exclusively pump. However, some will not understand why you don't just breastfeed and some won't understand why you don't just feed formula. Both opinions can be frustrating and difficult to tolerate, especially if you are already under stress.

For those people who want you to feed formula, simply explain the benefits of breast milk and explain how you want to provide the very best for your baby. Suggest that they too no doubt want the best for your child and you are thankful that now, having this information, they will support your decision. Do not give them the option to continue with their former position. Often comments such as theirs are not so much unsupportive of your pumping as they are concerned about you and the amount of time and effort they see you putting into pumping.

Sometimes people also fall victim to the overwhelming advertising from formula companies that often claim formula to be close to mother's milk. They need to be educated about breast milk. Many older adults also fed their children formula as babies and do not want to suggest that they perhaps did not provide the best for their children. It is often hard to look beyond your own situation, but by doing so you can often see where others are coming from.

For those people who think you should be breastfeeding, it is often more difficult to sway their opinion. Some simply don't understand why you would choose to pump even though for many women it is not a choice they wanted to make. People often don't recognize the exclusively pumping mother as having made a better choice than feeding formula. And some critics see exclusively pumping as second rate to breastfeeding and may say you are doing your baby a disservice. They may feel that every woman can breastfeed if they truly want to.

Regardless of a person's stance, all you can do is explain your position: why you are not breastfeeding and why you chose to exclusively pump instead of feed formula. Be understanding of how they may feel threatened by your dedication and determination, especially if they fed formula to their baby. Recognize most people's intentions are good. They may not realize how emotional it can be for you right now.

Here are a few thoughts on maintaining a strong relationship with friends and family:

- Explain that a happy, healthy baby makes you happy and healthy and also that their support and friendship will make it easier for you to continue.

- Avoid, as much as possible, those people who continue to be negative or outwardly unsupportive of your decision- it can be easy to give in to the will of others.

- Stay focused on your goals and let those around you know what your goals are so they can help you to achieve them.

- Become as mobile as possible. Some people may simply wish they could see more of you and feel that your pumping is taking away your ability to visit them or do things with them.

- Build new support systems when needed. Reach out into your community for new mothers programs, play groups, church groups, or La Leche League meetings.

Maintaining a Strong Relationship with Your Spouse

Simply adding a new baby into your life can be enough to turn your relationship with your spouse upside-down. Regardless of whether this is your first baby or not, adding a new life into your world takes some adjustment. Many men find it difficult to fit into the baby's world and see mothers as the ones who know everything: what to do and what's going on. It is important to involve your spouse as much as possible into the baby's daily activities, both for his benefit, the baby's benefit, and your own benefit.

Most spouses simply want their wife to be okay and seeing their wife stressed and exhausted and possibly in pain from a poor breastfeeding experience or pumping can be very concerning. This concern can sometimes manifest itself as being unsupportive of pumping. They may suggest a switch to formula not because they are unsupportive or do not want their baby to receive breast milk, but because they see how difficult it is for their wife. While some husbands are unsupportive, most are incredibly supportive and simply want their wife to be okay.

Share with your spouse the value of breast milk for both you and your baby. Enlist him to help educate family and friends; a united front can go a long way in swaying unsupportive family members. Also, share with your spouse the emotions you are feeling because of not being able to breastfeed. Often men find it difficult to recognize how strong a new mother's emotions are and do not realize how emotional the act of breastfeeding can be. Help him to understand this as best you can. Explain to him how his unwavering support is absolutely necessary for you to be successful exclusively pumping.

Suggest ways your spouse can support and assist you in making things easier such as:

- Cleaning bottles and your pump kit
- Caring for your older children
- Bathing the baby
- Feeding the baby
- Allowing you to relax and perhaps giving a back rub or foot rub
- Not mentioning weaning or feeding formula unless you have introduced the subject
- Being flexible and understanding your time is not as free as it once was
- Taking care of the household chores that you are unable to do easily such as outside work, grocery shopping, banking, and cooking the occasional dinner
- And whatever else you feel would support your ability to be successful exclusively pumping!

Some other things to consider:

- Talk to your spouse when you are pumping. Often this might be the only uninterrupted one-on-one time you will get during a day.

- Understand how you may feel differently about your body after having a baby as well as while you are breastfeeding/pumping. Share this with your spouse.

- Take advantage of people offering to babysit in order to spend some time with your spouse.

- Don't place expectations on your relationship. Understand it will evolve and change. Be flexible and patient and, most of all, have a sense of humour!

- Find support with other couples and mothers and talk with them about changes in their relationships.

- Lactation changes hormone levels in your body which can affect you in many ways. You may have a reduced sex drive and may experience vaginal dryness. These may not normalize until after you have weaned. You may want to speak to your doctor if they are particularly troublesome.

Exclusively Pumping Breast Milk

Weaning

When to Wean

When to wean is entirely your decision. The benefits of breast milk continue as long as you choose to feed it; however, it is more difficult to exclusively pump into the toddler years simply because of the demands it places on you. While some women are able to drop down to only two pumps a day and produce enough breast milk to meet the needs of their baby, these women are not the majority. For these women, continuing past a year is more feasible, but most women who are exclusively pumping wean around their baby's first birthday or earlier.

Your decision to wean will likely take into account a number of elements: your long-term goal, your baby's health, your health, your family, your emotions, your work requirements, and a number of other individual factors. In many cases, the decision to wean is a gradual one. You will perhaps feel that it is time and will take a few weeks to test the waters and try to gauge just how you feel about the idea of no longer feeding your baby your breast milk.

Do take the time to make the decision. Once you start the process of weaning, it is difficult (but not impossible) to reverse it. Make the decision based on your needs but also based on your emotions. Many mothers feel they need to wean due to their personal situation, but emotionally they are unwilling to give it up. Do not discount your emotions and make a purely intellectual decision.

Consider why you want to wean. If you are feeling overwhelmed, perhaps simply dropping a pumping session will make enough of a difference and you will decide to continue pumping. If your supply is the issue, get advice on how to increase it. Read the suggestions in the previous chapter "The Fundamentals of Exclusively Pumping". Be informed. Ensure you are confident that you have tried everything you are willing to try. Whatever your reasons, ensure that you are comfortable with your decision. Most women will feel at peace with their decision when it is the right time.

Guilt Associated With Weaning

Many women report feelings of guilt when they are considering weaning. However, most women are able to move beyond these feelings and settle into an understanding that the time is right to wean, recognizing that their feelings of guilt are more closely related to a sadness that they will no longer be providing breast milk for their baby. Some level of guilt or sadness is perhaps unavoidable and is also common in breastfeeding women. However, if you are feeling a tremendous, overwhelming sense of guilt, you need to investigate where these feelings are coming from.

Perhaps you are not yet ready to wean. Possibly you are weaning because of pressure to do so from friends or family members. Maybe you are weaning because you are returning to work and do not feel you can continue to pump when working. Perhaps you need to start a medication and have been told it is contraindicated while breastfeeding. In all these cases, perhaps you should continue to pump.

If you are simply not prepared to stop pumping and want to continue feeding your baby breast milk, then do so. Drop a session, alter your work load, or enlist the help of friends and family. Do whatever it takes to continue until you feel it is the right time to wean.

If your family or friends are pressuring you to wean, ignore them. Do what you want to do. It is your body and your baby. You are doing what you know is best for your child and you will also wean when you know it is best for you and your child.

If you are returning to work, there is no reason you need to wean. Employers are becoming more and more supportive of breastfeeding mothers and many large companies are even establishing pumping rooms and supplying fridges to store expressed breast milk. Speak to your employer about your needs to see if you can work out an arrangement. While it may require a little more effort and planning on your part, it is possible to work and pump.

If you need to start a new medication and are concerned about the possible effects to your baby, seek expert advice. Visit www.motherisk.org or Dr. Thomas Hale's site http://neonatal.ttuhsc.edu/lact/. While some medications are clearly not compatible with breastfeeding, some have minimal risks to the baby and, through careful consultation with your doctor and your child's doctor, you may decide it is beneficial for your baby to continue to receive breast milk and that the risk is acceptable. Or you may be able to find an alternative drug therapy that will not impact your breast milk. Do not wean until you are entirely satisfied that you have learned about all your options.

Making the Switch to Formula or Whole Cow's Milk

It is important to have a feeding plan for your baby in place before you start to wean (or at least before your freezer stash runs out if you are fortunate enough to have one). Speak with your baby's doctor about the best replacement for breast milk. Depending on your baby's requirements, you may need to consider specialty formulas or you may be able to switch to whole cow's milk if your baby is old enough and eating a wide variety of solids. Your child's doctor will be able to provide advice specific to your baby's requirements.

Many women become concerned that their baby may not accept the new food: whether it is formula or cow's milk. If you plan on switching to formula, you may feel more comfortable starting the weaning process if you know your baby will accept formula. Offer a bottle or two and see what happens. Many babies don't even notice there is something different in their bottle, and if this is the case for your child, it can make you more comfortable with the thought of weaning. When switching over to formula, do it gradually. Ask your child's doctor for their recommendation of how best to do it.

If your baby is not accepting of formula, you may want to consider slowly introducing the formula by mixing it with expressed breast milk. This slow introduction should also be done with whole cow's milk. Offer your baby's regular bottles mixed with one ounce of the formula or cow's milk.

Wait a day or two and then add another ounce while reducing the amount of breast milk. Watch your baby for any signs that the cow's milk or formula is not being tolerated well. Continue to add more formula or cow's milk and reduce the amount of expressed breast milk. Within a week or two, the substitution should be completed.

How to Wean

The process of weaning is actually quite simple and relates directly to how your supply is established and maintained. What you will be doing is everything you have avoided while you have been pumping, and you will be starting to do the things you were warned not to do.

Allow yourself enough time to do a slow, gradual wean. Do not expect to be finished on a set date. Instead, allow your body to dictate the schedule. The slower you wean, the fewer negative effects you will have from it. By slowly weaning, you can have a comfortable and easy end to your pumping experience.

Most women will only be pumping three or four times a day when they decide to wean. If you are pumping more, it will take longer for you to go through the process. Review, if necessary, how milk is produced and what processes are in place that maintain or increase supply. During weaning, you will be leaving milk in your breasts instead of removing as much as you usually would. This will signal your body to slow down and eventually stop production. You will also start to lengthen the time between pumping sessions.

The Process:

- The first step is to begin reducing the length of time you are pumping each session. Do not dramatically cut your sessions; instead, start by reducing the time you pump by only three to five minutes.

- See how your body responds.

- After a couple days, continue to reduce the length of your pumping sessions. Once again, only decrease the time by a couple minutes.

- You should start to see a small decline in your supply simply by reducing the length of time you are pumping.

- Continue to slowly reduce the length of sessions; ensure no hard spots or blocked ducts develop.

- Your next step is to begin stretching the amount of time between your pumping sessions as you would if you wanted to drop a pumping session. However, your goal is to eventually eliminate all sessions, so it is easiest not to get overly concerned about your pumping schedule by trying to pump at specific times. Instead, let your body start to guide you as to when you need to pump. Do not pump immediately when you start to feel full, instead wait until you feel you need to pump. Do not allow your breasts to become overly engorged, but do stretch out the time within comfortable limits.

- As you continue to reduce the length of your pumping sessions, you will see your supply decreasing and be able to go longer between pumps.

- Switch from a scheduled pumping regime to only pumping when you feel you need to. When you start to feel pressure or get engorged, pump. If you feel any hard spots developing, pump.

- If you are prone to blocked ducts or mastitis, take the weaning process very slowly! Do not allow yourself to get engorged. Pump to relieve the pressure as soon as it starts to develop, but do not pump to "empty" unless this is the only way to remove a block.

- The key at this stage is to only pump to relieve any hardness in your breasts. You *must* leave milk in your breasts. This is the only way to wean.

- Depending on how many pumping sessions you were doing when you started to wean, you will most likely see a dramatic decrease in your supply when you drop to around two sessions a day. Every woman is different though, so do not worry if your weaning experience is different than someone else's experience. Simply ensure that you are reducing the amount of time you are pumping and lengthening the time between pumping sessions. Stay focused on your weaning plan and don't be in a hurry to finish.

- Eventually you will get to a point where you only need to pump once a day and then you will be able to go thirty-six hours and then forty-eight hours and then you will perhaps be able to go five or even seven days before needing to pump again.

- Most women, once they have weaned to this point, find that they do need to pump at least once after a week or so. If you are having any tenderness or pressure in your breasts, it is best to pump for a very short time- five or ten minutes- just to relieve the discomfort. This usually is the last time you will need to pump.

- Your breasts will continue to produce small amounts of milk for several weeks, or even months, and if you try, you will be able to hand express small drops. Eventually, this too will end.

If you start to wean from two or three pumping sessions a day, you can expect the process to take approximately two to three weeks.

Relief for Engorgement and Discomfort

It should be your goal during the weaning process to avoid engorgement and discomfort; however, it may be impossible in every case. If you do experience any soreness or engorgement, try the following suggestions to relieve your discomfort:

- Use cold compresses to relieve the swelling. Do not use hot compresses since this will only make the situation worse.

- Use a pain reliever such as acetaminophen or ibuprofen.

- Wear a supportive, well-fitting bra but do *not* wear one with an underwire and do *not* bind your breasts since this can encourage blocked ducts to develop.

- Try putting chilled, green cabbage leaves in your bra for approximately 20 minutes several times a day.

- Try using herbs such as dried sage, jasmine, peppermint, spearmint, lemon balm, or oregano to reduce your milk supply. See the following web page for further information about using herbs:

  http://www.kellymom.com/herbal/milksupply/herbs-oversupply.html

- You may have avoided the use of hormonal birth control while pumping, but it is okay to start using them now. They may cause a reduction in your supply.

- The decongestant pseudoephedrine found in numerous over-the-counter cold and allergy medications can, as one of its side-effects, reduce milk supply. It is passed through breast milk though.

- Most importantly, go slowly! You should have very little, if any, discomfort when weaning.

The After-Effects of Weaning

Once you have weaned, give yourself time to adjust to your new life. It can feel very unusual no longer having your time strictly scheduled. Enjoy your regained freedom and take some time to reflect on your accomplishment.

Once you have weaned, your period should return if it has not already. It may take a few months for your cycle to normalize. And you may find that you have heavier periods than before you were pregnant. This is completely normal.

After weaning, you may find that your breasts are smaller than their pre-pregnancy size. This is also normal since the milk producing glands replaced the fatty tissue in the breasts during lactation. The fat will return and your breasts should return to a similar size as before.

You may also find that your emotions are much more on edge as your hormone levels return to their normal state. During lactation, your estrogen levels are very low and once you wean they will return to their pre-pregnancy state.

Your appetite may also change. Often it will decrease. You may need to be more careful about what you are eating since it will be much easier to gain weight now that you are no longer expending the extra energy required to produce milk.

In general, give yourself time to relax and reflect on your experience exclusively pumping. No doubt you have seen the benefits of your decision in your baby, and you will continue to see them for years to come. It is an experience that rarely leaves a woman unchanged. You have most likely grown and recognized the strength you have inside of you to do whatever you feel is best for you and your family. Enjoy your baby; he won't be a baby for long! Best wishes to you and your family and congratulations on choosing to give your baby the best gift possible: mother's milk.

Resources

Support Groups and Discussion Boards

http://bbs.babycenter.com/board/baby/babybreastfeed/1
202053
- BabyCenter Discussion Board- Pumping Moms. For all mothers who are pumping, not just exclusive pumpers.

http://messageboards.ivillage.com/iv-ppexcluspump
- iVillage Exclusively Pumping Discussion Board. An extremely active board.

http://groups.yahoo.com/group/EPers/
- Yahoo! Discussion Group for women who are exclusively pumping.

http://health.groups.yahoo.com/group/PumpMoms/
- Yahoo! Pumpmoms Discussion Group. For all mothers who are pumping, not just exclusive pumpers.

http://health.groups.yahoo.com/group/mobi/
- Mothers Overcoming Breastfeeding Issues. A discussion group dedicated to women who are coming to terms with not being able to successfully breastfeed.

http://bbs.babycenter.com/board/baby/babyfeeding/1379
847
- Unable to Breastfeed Board at BabyCenter

http://messageboards.ivillage.com/iv-pppumpends
- When Pumping Ends discussion board at iVillage

General Breastfeeding/Pumping Information

http://www.infactcanada.ca/InfactHomePage.htm
- INFACT Canada. An organization dedicated to the protection, promotion and support of breastfeeding.

http://www.breastfeeding.co.uk/index.html
- Jane's Breastfeeding Resource

http://www.breastfeedingonline.com
- Breastfeeding Online. An excellent collection of breastfeeding and lactation information.

http://bflrc.com
- Bright Futures Lactation Resource Center. An good collection of information for breastfeeding and lactation

www.kellymom.com
- Excellent information on breastfeeding and attachment parenting.

http://www.promom.org/
- ProMom is a non-profit organization dedicated to increasing public awareness and public acceptance of breastfeeding.

http://www.lalecheleague.org/home_intro.html
- La Leche League. Excellent information for breastfeeding and lactation as well as connections to breastfeeding support in your community.

http://www.pumpingmoms.org/
- Web site maintained by Pumpmoms listserv

http://pages.ivillage.com/epers/
- Web site maintained by Exclusively Pumping discussion board at iVillage

http://www.thebirthden.com
- Site includes articles written by Dr. Jack Newman as well as informative video clips to assist with breastfeeding.

Breast Pump Manufacturers and Information

http://www.ameda.com/
- Ameda Breast Pumps and Supplies

http://www.aventbaby.com/uk/index.asp
- Avent Breast Pumps, Bottles, and Accessories

http://www.baileymed.com/
- Bailey Medical Engineering Nurture III Breast Pump

http://www.whittlestone.com/
- Whittlestone Breast Pump

http://www.whisperwear.com/
- Whisper Wear Breast Pump

http://www.medela.com/
- Medela Breast Pumps and Supplies

http://www.ameda.com/products/new_study.htm
- Ameda's hygenikit claims

http://www.breastfeedingonline.com/pumps.shtml
- Information on used breast pumps

http://www.leron-line.com/updates/Breast_Pumps.htm
- Information on breast pumps

http://www.medela.com/NEWFILES/faq/preownpump.html
- Information from Medela about used breast pumps

http://www.artofbreastfeeding.com/cgi-bin/store/AoB2.cgi?CPAGE=Choosing.html
- Information on choosing the right breast pump for your situation

http://www.artofbreastfeeding.com/cgi-bin/store/AoB2.cgi?ORDER_ID=107261715354&CPAGE=used.html
- Information on using a pre-owned breast pump

http://www.expectantmothersguide.com/library/pittsburgh/EPGbreastpump.htm
- Information on choosing the right breast pump

Articles about Exclusively Pumping

http://www.lalecheleague.org/llleaderweb/LV/LVFebMar01p3.html
- "Supporting the Human Milk Feeding Mother" by Jill Landis

http://www.drspock.com/faq/0,1511,3772,00.html
- "Ask Our Expert- Pumping Instead of Nursing"

http://www.medela.com/NewFiles/exclusivepumpg.html
- Medela article on Exclusively Pumping by Kathleen B. Bruce

http://www.parentsplace.com/babies/bfeed/articles/0,,16 6427_251068,00.html
- Article about Exclusively Pumping from Parents Place

http://www.bflrc.com/ljs/breastfeeding/bfnotwk.htm
- "Long-Term Pumping When Breastfeeding Doesn't Work Out" by Linda J. Smith

http://www.artofbreastfeeding.com/pump2.html
- "Women Who Forgo Breastfeeding for Pumping" by Nancy Mohrbacher

http://www.ivillage.com/topics/pregbaby/0,,166427,00.ht ml
- Pumping Breast Milk articles at iVillage

http://www.canadianparents.com/articles/feature85d.htm
- An article about the loss and sadness of not being able to breastfeed

http://breastfeed.com/resources/articles/bottlefilled.htm
- "A Bottle Filled With Breast Milk" by Krissi Danielsson

http://www.mother-2-mother.com/ExclusivePumping.htm
- A good article with the basics of exclusively pumping

http://members.aol.com/KBone91/pumping.html
- An article about exclusively pumping for preemies focusing on the emotional aspect.

Breast Milk and the Benefits of Breastfeeding

http://www.hc-sc.gc.ca/pphb-dgspsp/rhs-ssg/factshts/brstfd_e.html
- Canadian Perinatal Surveillance Survey

http://www.statcan.ca/english/freepub/82-221-XIE/00503/nonmed/behaviours4.htm
- Health Indicators from Statistics Canada

http://www.hc-sc.gc.ca/dca-dea/publications/pdf/reasons_to_bf_e.pdf
- "10 Great Reasons to Breastfeed" by Health Canada

http://www.paho.org/English/HPP/HPN/Benefits_of_BF.htm
- Benefits of Breastfeeding from the Pan American Health Organization

http://medicalreporter.health.org/tmr0297/breastfeed0297.html
- "Breastfeeding: Good for Babies, Mothers, and the Planet" by Dr. Alicia Dermer and Dr. Anne Montgomery

http://www.medscape.com/viewarticle/408813
- "Breastfeeding: Unraveling Mysteries of Mother's Milk" by Margit Hamosh, PhD

http://www.promom.org/bf_info/sci_am.htm
- "How Breast Milk Protects Newborns" by Dr. Jack Newman

http://www.bflrc.com/ljs/breastfeeding/shakenot.htm
- "Don't Shake the Milk" by Linda J. Smith

http://www.bflrc.com/ljs/breastfeeding/MakeMilk.html
- "How Mother's Milk is Made" by Linda J. Smith

http://hometown.aol.com/davisrnclc/myhomepage/how.htm
- "Anatomy of How the Breast Makes Milk" by Marie Davis

http://www.emedicine.com/ped/topic2594.htm
- "Human Milk and Lactation" by Carol L. Wagner, MD

http://www.hc-sc.gc.ca/dca-dea/publications/pdf/infant_e.pff
- "Nutrition for Healthy Term Infants" by the Canadian Pediatrics Society, Dieticians of Canada, and Health Canada

http://www.kellymom.com/bf/supply/milkproduction.html
- "How Does Milk Production Work?" from Kellymom.com

http://www.saanendoah.com/compare.html
- "Comparing Milk: Human, Cow, Goat & Commercial Infant Formula" compiled by Stephanie Clark, Ph. D

http://www.medela.com/NewFiles/faq/benefitsbfdg.html
- "Benefits of Breastfeeding" from Medela

Storage and Handling of Breast Milk

http://www.lalecheleague.org/FAQ/milkstorage.html
- Milk storage information from La Leche League

http://breastfeeding.hypermart.net/storagehandling.html
- Storage and handling of expressed breast milk

http://www.lalecheleague.org/NB/NBJulAug98p109.html
- Information on storing expressed breast milk

http://www.breastfeed-essentials.com/storagehandling.html
- Storing and handling expressed breast milk

http://www.askdrsears.com/html/2/t026900.asp#T02690
1
- Storing and handling expressed breast milk from Dr.
  Sears

http://www.medela.com/NewFiles/faq/coll_store.html
- Information on storing and handling expressed breast
  milk from Medela

http://www.latrobe.edu.au/microbiology/milk.html
- Tables of antimicrobial factors and microbiological
  contaminants relevant to human milk banking from La
  Trobe University

Common Concerns (including concerns about supply)

http://www.breastfeedingonline.com/22.html
- Blocked ducts and mastitis

http://www.breastfeedingonline.com/candidaprotocol.html
- Dr. Jack Newman's yeast/thrush protocol

http://www.breastfeedingonline.com/20.html
- Information on using Fluconazole Diflucan

http://www.bflrc.com/ljs/breastfeeding/dryupfst.htm
- Information on rapid weaning

http://www.breastfeedingonline.com/24.html
- Miscellaneous treatments from Dr. Jack Newman

http://www.leron-line.com/updates/wound_healing.htm
- Information on moist wound healing

http://www.breastfeedingonline.com/3b.html
- Treatment for sore nipples

http://www.breastfeedingonline.com/6.html
- Using gentian violet

http://www.lalecheleague.org/ba/May99.html
- "Cue feeding: wisdom and science" by Lisa Marasco and Jan Barger

http://www.bflrc.com/newman/breastfeeding/domperid.htm
- Information on using Domperidone

http://www.breastfeedingonline.com/fenuhugg-print.html
- Information on using Fenugreek

http://www.rcrh.org/Services/Lactation/Teaching.asp
- Information on using Reglan

http://www.kellymom.com/bf/concerns/mom/mastitis.html
- Information about blocked ducts and mastitis

http://www.kellymom.com/nutrition/vitamins/lecithin.html
- Information on using lecithin for blocked ducts

http://www.kellymom.com/bf/concerns/mom/recurrent-mastitis.html
- Information on recurrent mastitis or blocked ducts

Products for Pumping

http://groups.yahoo.com/group/PM_BSFT/
- This is a new Yahoo! group for women who wish to sell, trade, or giveaway supplies related to breastfeeding and pumping. Please use caution and inform yourself of the warnings against using previously used personal use breast pumps. However, there are many items that can safely and easily be sterilized for reuse.

http://www.expressyourselfmums.co.uk
- A company in the UK that focuses on the needs of women who are breastfeeding or expressing breast milk.

Note: There are many online stores that sell breast pumps and supplies- far too many to list here. A quick web search will provide you with a large number of retailers. Also, ask women on the discussion boards for their recommendation of suppliers. Internet retailers usually seem to offer pumps at lower prices than most bricks and mortar stores. Check around! Be careful of eBay offerings, however, since there is little protection for you if you buy a new pump from someone and it ends up not being new. Also, there have been reports of people selling stolen rental pumps through online auctions. If in doubt, get a serial number and call the pump manufacturer.

Miscellaneous Sites

http://www.fda.gov/bbs/topics/ANSWERS/2004/ANS012 92.html
- FDA warning against the use of domperidone

http://www.askdrsears.com/html/5/t051100.asp
- Information about baby wearing by Dr. Sears

http://www.nineinnineout.org
- Nine in Nine Out Babywearing Organization

http://www.hmbana.com
- Human Milk Banking Association of North America

http://www.ukamb.org/
- United Kingdom Association for Milk Banking

http://www.motherisk.org/
- Information about the safety and risk of drugs during pregnancy and breastfeeding

http://neonatal.ttuhsc.edu/lact/index.html
- Breastfeeding Pharmacology site by Dr. Thomas Hale

http://www.drjaygordon.com/bf/worknursetips.htm
- Information about working/nursing/pumping

http://www.kangaroomothercare.com
- Dr. Nils Bergman on the importance kangaroo mother care (KMC)

http://peach.ease.lsoft.com/archives/lactnet.html
- Archives of LACTNET; a listserv for lactation professionals. While not directed at pumping, you can find some useful information about lactation issues.

http://home.vicnet.net.au/%7Eearlyed/oct/oexpress.htm
- Article directed specifically at pumping for a premature baby

http://www.bflrc.com/newman/breastfeeding/guilt.htm
- "Breastfeeding and Guilt" by Dr. Jack Newman

http://biochem.uwa.edu.au/PEH/PEHRes.html
- Professor Peter Hartmann is a leading researcher in human lactation. This is a site discussing his research.

http://www.ilca.org
- International Lactation Consultant Association

Additional Resources

Alm, B. et al (2002). Breast feeding and the sudden infant death syndrome in Scandinavia, 1992-95 [Electronic version]. *Arch Dis Child*, 86, 400-402.

American Academy of Pediatrics (1997). Breastfeeding and the use of human milk [Electronic version]. *Pediatrics*, 100(6), 1035-1039.

British Medical Association. (2003, December). Saving expressed breast milk [Electronic version]. *British Medical Journal*, 327(7427), 1338-1.

Deodhar, L., Joshi, S. (1991). Microbiological study of breast milk with special reference to its storage in milk bank [Electronic version]. *Journal of Postgraduate Medicine*, 37 (1), 14-6.

Hanson, Lars (1998, December). Breastfeeding provides passive and likely long-lasting active immunity [Electronic version]. *Annals of Allergy, Asthma, & Immunology*, 81, 523-37.

Jones, E., Dimmock, P. W., & Spencer, S. A. (2001, September). A randomized controlled trial to compare methods of milk expression after preterm delivery [Electronic version]. *Arch Dis Child Fetal Neonatal Ed.* 85, F91-F95.

Resources